# Perfect
# Pause

# Perfect Pause

A Woman's Guide to Preventing
Weight Gain, Aging Gracefully and Living
Her Best Life Through Menopause

## DR. GOLDWYN B. FOGGIE

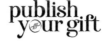

Published by Publish Your Gift®
An imprint of Purposely Created Publishing Group, LLC

Scriptures marked ESV are taken from English Standard Version®. Copyright © 2001 by Crossway, a publishing ministry of Good News Publishers. All rights reserved.

Scriptures marked KJV are taken from the Holy Bible, King James Version. All rights reserved.

Printed in the United States of America

ISBN: 978-1-64484-583-7 (print)
ISBN: 978-1-64484-584-4 (ebook)

Special discounts are available on bulk quantity purchases by book clubs, associations and special interest groups. For details email: sales@publishyourgift.com or call (888) 949-6228. For information log on to www.PublishYourGift.com

# Dedication

This book is dedicated to all you preoccupied profession-als, midlife mamas, and board-room bosses keeping it all together while going through the change of life. It will as-sist women to embrace the changes in their bodies and navigate a healthier perspective as they encounter meno-pause and all the changes that go along with it, especially the hormonal changes which contribute to the dreaded weight gain and unflattering fluffiness. Ladies, we can age amazingly and find time for ourselves so that we don't fall to pieces. After all, we are the ones that everybody depends on. Although we inspire and care for others, we deserve to pour into ourselves and preserve our sexiness. Keep that in mind as you read the chapters of this book. I've discovered what works for me, and I'm excited to share it with you. So, let's pause—perfectly—to step into this next phase of life with patience, perfection, and pizazz!

# **Table of Contents**

# When Menopause Comes Knocking at Your Door

"What is happening to my body?" you might be asking.

What isn't happening is the better question. Have you noticed that your body is going through so many unwanted changes as a result of menopause and the process of aging that you can hardly keep up with them? It seems like almost every aspect of your life as you know it is changing. From an increase in sagging skin to changes in vision. From hearing loss to constipation. From W.A.P. to now feeling like the Sahara. And those aching knees seemed to come out of nowhere.

One of the biggest obstacles I see women face as a weight loss doctor, is their battle of the bulge. The unending difficulty of trying to fit into their clothes without having to buy larger sizes. The challenge of keeping the fat on the back of your arms from flapping in the wind and the difficulty of watching your once svelte waistline expand over your belt line is just agonizing. No one escapes all the effects of aging, but most of us would sure as hell like to slow them down just a wee bit. And we'd like to avoid the changes which result in us having to suck in our middles and turn to the side when posing for pictures on the 'gram. Ladies, let's be honest: We'd like to minimize the unappealing signs of aging. But most of all, we'd like to stay as independent and productive as possible as we can for as long as we can and as God sees fit.

This book is my blueprint to help you to live your best life as you strive to age as beautifully and gracefully and shed those dreadfully unwanted pounds that seem to be creeping up on your thighs and your belly like a thief in the night. If your struggle with weight has gone from *Oh, I'm just trying to stay in shape* to *OH MY GOD! Body, why hath thou forsaken me? This can't possibly be my body that is staring back at me in the mirror! Where is this fat coming from?* I'm going to let you in on a little secret. It's not too late for you, my midlife mavens. I don't care if you've been struggling with weight your entire life. You can beat this. You can lose those unwanted pounds that seem to find you, especially during this time of your life.

I know because I've been dodging fat cells and that dreaded menopausal pooch and cellulite for the past five years. I feel I've found the secret formula to staying slim and aging gracefully—and I'm going to help you do it as well. And you know what, divas? It's not as difficult as you think it is.

Thankfully, this is the time in our lives that we have been waiting for. We can finally do some of the things we have always wanted to do and go to the places we've always dreamed about. Most of us are emptying out the nest and embracing life with a *carpe diem* attitude. And guess what? We don't have to work out hours and hours every day to maintain our figures. We don't have to starve ourselves and never eat our favorite dessert or forgo a nice glass of wine. Are you ready for it?

Healthy aging is defined by the World Health Organization (WHO) as the process of developing and maintaining the functional ability that enables wellbeing in older age. As described by the WHO, our ability to age healthfully encompasses being able to meet our basic needs, which includes learning and growing and making decisions for ourselves, remaining mobile while building and maintaining relationships, and finally, to continue to be productive members of society.

This growing older conundrum comes with a boat load of unwelcome changes, I'll admit. As our moods begin to shift, due to either the sudden or gradual decline in sex hormone production by the ovaries, particularly estrogen, women may experience a multitude of symptoms that seem to wreak havoc on our bodies. Let's talk about it. Aging well together. Who am I kidding? I don't want to only age well, I want to hold my place as being the absolute baddest bitch in the room! You feel me? Let's get to it. But first, let me introduce you to a few of the most common menopausal conundrums women face:

## HOT FLUSHES

We may have vasomotor symptoms in response to a decrease in estrogens called hot flushes. These personal summers are best described as waves of heat that well up on the inside of the body and coalesce into beads of sweat that appear on the face, neck, and chest. It's as if an internal flame ignites inside the body. And the need to cool off instantly becomes your number one priority.

## SLEEPING ISSUES

Sleeping, which once had been regular and effortless, starts to become more interrupted and less frequent. Sometimes due to the abrupt hot flashes through the night and the need to empty the bladder more often, we find ourselves practically up and down all throughout the night. We transition into nocturnal creatures in our homes while the world sleeps and suddenly we are not ourselves anymore. Issues with urination are also linked to the lack of estrogen in the genitourinary tract and may manifest as an increased urge to go to the bathroom. Urination may also be more painful and frequent urinary tract infections can occur, which can make sleep feel impossible.

Sometimes you may not know why sleep escapes you, but when you don't get enough, the next day you feel fatigued, have brain fog, and a notice the sheer lack of energy required to get you through your normal day. This tiredness becomes chronic when night after night your sleep is both interrupted and inadequate.

## VAGINAL ATROPHY

Vaginal atrophy—another term for vaginal dryness—caused by thinning of the lining of the vaginal epithelium may start to occur. This is most often recognized during moments of intimacy when you find yourself in the throes of passion and you suddenly—and most unexpectantly—experience vaginal dryness and discomfort. Or you are getting ready for an intimate moment, but your vagina thinks differently and isn't even trying to join the party. I mean, WTF? This reminds me of the same feeling you get when you accidentally wash your favorite sweater instead of sending it to the dry cleaners and it shrinks two sizes. You then try to stuff your size large body in that size small sweater. You know it's too tight. And it's uncomfortable. But you keep trying to wear that sweater because you've been wearing it forever and it's your favorite. You keep thinking, "I really love that sweater!" Now you contort and stretch yourself to get in that sweater just to prove a point.

## WEIGHT GAIN

Gaining weight is a common yet annoying symptom of menopause that no one likes. The appearance of increased body fat is noticed when your clothes are suddenly feeling tighter and more uncomfortable. Your Coke-bottle figure is starting to look more rectangular, like SpongeBob SquarePants. Thick in the middle and no matter what you eat, fat tends to find you. As my friend Aubree says, fat doesn't ever take a vacation! Most of my clients in my practice are middle-aged women, somewhere between the ages of forty and sixty. They come to me because they are experiencing gradual, unwanted weight gain—twenty, thirty, or even fifty pounds. It sometimes seems to appear out of nowhere. And other times, it slowly creeps up on them. The typical complaint I hear is "Dr. Goldie, I'm gaining a lot of weight, but I hardly eat anything. I don't understand why I'm gaining weight?" They don't feel like themselves. They don't like the changes they see in the mirror, and they want to see a change as quickly as possible.

There are more than a few reasons why weight gain happens. The decrease in sex hormone production, results in the adipose (fat) cells attempting to make more estrogen by producing more and more fat cells. This typically occurs in the visceral fat located in the midsection where no woman wants to pick up extra weight. Visceral body fat is the fat that's stored deep inside the belly. It's deposited around the organs including the liver and the intestines. This is the hidden fat which makes the belly stick out and gives the body an apple shaped appearance. Excess visceral fat is unhealthy because visceral fat makes hormones and chemicals that are toxic to the body and increases the risks of diseases such as: osteoarthritis, asthma, liver disease, cancer, cardiovascular disease, and dementia. The best way to reduce visceral fat is by changing your diet and exercising. Disappointingly, liposuction does not get rid of this type of fat, ladies.

Additionally, as we age, we are steadily losing muscles cells which leads to the constant slowing down of our metabolism. Missing work outs and losing lean muscle is a recipe for an increase of fat cells. During middle age we typically lose up to 3 percent of muscle cells per year. This is called sarcopenia, which is caused by an imbalance of signals that control muscle growth versus muscle break down. Sarcopenia limits our ability to perform many of our routine daily activities. What types of changes in our activities might we see as we age? We hire a landscaper instead of mowing the lawn ourselves. We take an Uber instead of taking the train to work and walking up a flight of stairs to the platform and three blocks from the train to our office. We order Instacart instead of carrying our own groceries in and out of the car. The less we do, the more limited we become, which will eventually shorten our life expectancy.

The great news is that menopausal weight gain is not inevitable. There are many things we can do to offset this and keep our weight in check. But we just have to be very strategic to prevent weight gain after menopause.

Identifying hurdles that slow down fat loss is key, as the Cleveland Clinic identified. Tracking your foods becomes important. It's also helpful to prioritize healthy calories and avoid skipping meals. But we'll get into more specifics later.

## MY STORY

I'd like to share more of my menopausal experience with you before I truly begin to show you how I've been able to limit my midlife weight gain and ward off the excess pounds. I'm here to reassure you that it absolutely can be done. You can successfully get through this midlife crisis and win the battle of the bulge.

Menopause hit me like a ton of bricks! When I turned fifty-one years old, I felt as if my body betrayed me and said "No ma'am. I don't think so." The activities that I previous enjoyed and was committed to, became incredibly difficult to engage in. Every day I would awaken with the goal of joining my running friends, but my body clearly rebelled and declared, "This is not going to happen!" My energy shifted greatly and my dedicated time to run with my friends became a past time. No matter how hard I tried, my body would not, could not get out of bed by 4:30 a.m. to make the 5:00 a.m. group runs. It was as if someone flipped a switch and zapped all the motivation out of my body to do what it had become very accustomed to doing for the past several years.

No matter what time I went to bed the night before or what time I got up, I simply lost my desire to get out of bed, get dressed, and drive to the park to run with my friends so early in the morning. Well, why were the runs so early you might ask? That was the time when we could all manage to get together for work outs before we had to go to work. Or before we had to go to school. How many of you have ever intended to do a workout or go to an exercise class or take a walk but get caught up in meetings or have to work late or take the kids to basketball practice? By the end of the day, you neglected to take time out for yourself. Then before you realize, its become a pattern.

Well, one week turned into one month. One month turned into one season then before I knew it, me and running had officially broken up and had not seen each other in over a year. This was devastating for me because running and I had been an item for many years. We were a couple. Running and I had innumerable rendezvous together. In the park, on the lakefront, through my neighborhood. Both privately and publicly. On training runs, trails, mud runs and obstacle course races. Through many seasons and occasions, running and I had become exclusive. We were tight as a grip. We had even made plans that one day we would spend 26.2 miles together in our first marathon, but now it seemed that this would never happen.

I had to come to the realization that at this time of my life, I had to shift some things around in my work schedule to a more amenable time to do my workouts. For me this became 7:00 a.m. awakenings instead of 4:30 a.m. and the start of incorporating more cross-training workouts to maintain my fitness which included spinning, weightlifting, and high intensity interval training. Sometimes you've got to pivot and change your approach to prioritizing your fitness. This became one example of me learning to pivot to stay fit. I've incorporated several other strategies to stay healthy throughout this phase of my life which so far have seem to be working well.

The cessation of estrogen production in my body has been an adjustment physically, hormonally, and emotionally. I've had to change some of my expectations and wishes I had held on to for time. Honestly, I'm figuring it out for myself, and it's finally working.

I've fine-tuned a game-plan for my life that I'd like to share with you in hopes that you too may benefit from what I've learned. This is my blueprint to assist you in living your best life as you too strive to lose weight and age beautifully. Embrace it. Let's age *backwards* together.

## CHAPTER 1

# Remove Your Barriers
# to Better Health

## MASTER YOUR MINDSET

Your decision to change your life begins and ends with you and the wonderful thoughts, dreams, and wishes that exist in your mind. Our minds are the most incredible, unbelievable, and—dare I say—powerful tool that God gave us to be the power centers of our bodies and behaviors. It's the conscious and unconscious part of the human brain which controls our every single thought. It's sort of the Grand Central Station of our physical forms. It tells our bodies what and what not to do. It helps us makes decisions good or bad by sending and receiving signals from our external world then interpreting them. Our minds set the tone for success or failure by controlling how we think, how we feel, and how we choose. When deciding to embark on a healthy lifestyle we toil with the reasons why we need to or don't need to do it. Why we should or should not do certain things and why we can or cannot make it happen. Some find this process very easy, yet others find it extremely difficult.

Why is this? There is a struggle that takes place between the mind and the body in most of these instances because our bodies want to be satisfied. We want to be comfortable and coddled in some cases and stimulated or satisfied in others. We don't want to be uncomfortable. We steer away from discomfort, fatigue, or stress. We steer away from the nagging feeling of hunger. We avoid displeasure at all costs. And when we fail to make healthy choices, it's usually because we want to do what our bodies want us to do. It's a tug of war going on between the mind and the body. A war of wills. The dilemma is who wins out on the battle of what one should do.

I am here to assure you that you can do what you set your mind to. You can go from couch potato to Pilates if you so choose. You can start in a twenty-six dress size and end in a size ten. Or you can dare to wear your size four dresses in your closet from med school through menopause without the assistance of Spanx, shape wear, girdles, binders, and the myriad of other undergarments that are out there to hold in, hide, mask, and disguise the fact that you are not in shape. And you can transform yourself from poor health to amazing potential. The possibilities are endless. I can confidently say this because I have witnessed the transformations multiple times in my patients, family members, and friends who I've assisted through my programs. It has been most rewarding. And it all started with me. My decision to change my life from worn out

OB/GYN physician to Wellness Warrior extraordinaire which changed the trajectory of my future.

## UTILIZE THE ADDITION EFFECT

Have you ever played the game Jenga? It's a fun game where wooden blocks are stacked in rows onto a tower and one by one a chosen block is removed and stacked on top of the tower. As each block is removed, it causes instability in the tower which contributes to the eventual overturn of the tower. The object of this game is to be the last successful player to remove and stack a block before a player makes the tower fall. Similarly, wellness is built by stacking one healthy decision onto the next onto the next with the goal of leading to a more balanced existence.

I began my health journey, which I fondly call my journey to wellness, years ago after my second child was a few years old. I had completed my residency and was practicing as a young attending. I joined the YMCA and attended aerobics class. From there, I realized how amazing it felt to participate regularly in fitness activities and I gradually added running then eventually swimming and biking. Little by little I found more activities to explore, but it did not happen overnight. It just felt good, and I liked feeling stronger and more energetic as time went on. I soon realized that exercise alone without eating right upsets the apple cart so to speak, and it didn't give me the results that I was seeking, so I began my attempt to better eating. This was the most difficult, as I had thirty years of habits and tendencies that I'd lived with and, in many ways, did not want to part with. I mean let's face it, we love what we love! I realized that I was a junk food junkie! I loved the taste of hamburgers and French fries and all the other food treats that contribute to obesity and tooth decay.

I can vividly remember being in the first grade, at lunch time sitting at my desk eating the lunch my mother had prepared for me from a brown paper bag while another student, Giselle, ate McDonald's for lunch because she forgot her sandwich at home. I was only six years of age and I recall the first time I smelled those fragrant French fries. I didn't want to eat a dry bologna sandwich. I wanted that hamburger and French fries. I craved the amazing combination of salt, sugar, and fat that most of us crave. Throughout my childhood, whenever I got the opportunity to eat outside the home, I wanted to do it. I loved sodas, chocolate milkshakes, and candy. Lots and lots of candy. It is no wonder that I spent an entire summer at the age of sixteen with my dentist getting cavities filled. I remember the sound of his drill in my mouth and the splatter of saliva hitting my face as he filled all six cavities in my mouth before I got my braces. I think I developed a slight crush on my dentist after all the time we spent being so close and all. Enjoying healthy foods was not on my radar. I had not been taught because my parents didn't understand the relationship between eating healthy food and maintaining a healthy body.

A healthy diet without adequate sleep won't give you your desired results. You also need to have proper rest to rejuvenate the body and shed excess pounds. When I don't get adequate sleep, my energy is too low. I'm less focused and I can't even think clearly. I certainly don't make the best food choices. A clear benefit of sleep is that it lowers inflammation which may lower the risk of heart disease. Some studies even suggest that lack of sleep may impair how glucose is processed therefore increase the risk of type 2 diabetes. Lack of sleep increases cortisol levels which increases stress to the body. We need to manage our sleep to optimize weight loss and improve metabolic health. I constantly struggled with sleep as an OB/GYN physician. It may not have been apparent in my outward appearance, but it showed up in my metabolic scores. I was exhibiting borderline blood pressures intermittently. Not high enough to initiate medications but not low enough to be considered normal. I always blamed it on something. I would say to myself maybe it's the blood pressure cuff. Or maybe it's because I didn't get enough sleep. Or perhaps I was under too much stress. Or maybe it's something I ate. Or it runs in my family, so I am predisposed to developing hypertension. Does any of this sound familiar? Have you ever said this to yourself? These are things we say when we're in denial. I needed a life change. I desperately needed a lifestyle makeover. Better sleep and stress management combined with healthful eating and exercise improved my scores tremendously.

Proper hydration is also a large piece of the puzzle of healthy habits. Without it your road to better health and ultimate weight loss is an uphill battle. I inadvertently trained my body to survive without drinking an adequate amount of water every day during residency training. As an intern, my day in the hospital began with pre-rounds on the patients at 5:00 a.m. before my senior resident made her appearance. Rounds were at 6:00 a.m. with her and the attending physician. Next, I dutifully transported patients to the O.R. on gurneys by 7:00 a.m. for surgery so that all surgeries could start on time. Then I had to write nursing orders and escort patients for routine tests all day, so that by the time my attending and senior resident completed their surgeries, I could update them on all the progress of the patients before evening rounds. On clinic days, after rounds we went to clinic and managed to see about 100 patients between us four residents before we went back to complete evening rounds and—hopefully—were able to go home.

I did not drink water because I did not want bathroom time to cut into my ability to get my tasks done for the day and this unhealthy habit followed me throughout four arduous years of OB/GYN residency. Water boosts our immune system. It aids in digestion. Poor hydration is the quickest way to become constipated. Water helps promote healthy skin by improving circulation through the capillaries. It helps us to flush out toxins from the body. Adequate water intake promotes satiety or fullness and, oftentimes, when we haven't had enough water and we think we're hungry we are actually thirsty and need to drink, not eat. This is how adequate water intake can help you lose more weight. Water can even fight bad breath by removing food particles from your mouth after eating.

Stress is also a huge excuse we use to avoid our goals. It can actually negatively impact your body, your mood, and your behavior. Stress triggers a flight or fight response in the body which puts you in a state of unrest which may increase the risks of disease. Emotional effects may include depression or anxiety. Physical effects resulting from lower immunity may increase the risks of more colds, flus, and even cardiovascular disease. Hormonal effects of increased stress can trigger reactions that increase hunger which trigger overeating and result in weight gain. My mom always used to say disease is caused by dis-ease. Studies confirm that many health problems are related to stress and certainly increase the risks of "dis-ease."

I found myself carrying ten to fifteen extra pounds on my frame just by being stressed. I've had to become better at managing it and walking away from situations that brought me excess stress. I've also become better at not caring about what people thought about it. I spent too many years caring about what people thought of me. The hilarious thing about it is that none of that matters. People don't spend their time thinking about my life or my decisions. Even if they did, why in the world should I care? I found out that people generally care about what you do as it relates to them. No one loses sleep about your life so why should you lose sleep about it.

A balanced life includes a combination of healthy habits stacked one on top another which we repeat over and over and over again. Once you start to create and maintain healthy habits, you'll notice a change in your body for the better.

## ELIMINATE YOUR EXCUSES

How many of us decide, I'm going to start working out? Yes. This time, I'm definitely going to start exercising at the gym. After all I'm paying a monthly membership and have not seen the inside of the gym since I joined? Okay well when am I going to start? How about Monday? You need to start your workout routine on Monday. Why Monday? Why can't you start today? Today is as good a day as any day, right? For some reason, Mondays are viewed as the day for starting over. Getting a fresh start. Getting motivated at the start of the new week helps us get over our weekend overindulgences. This is the same concept that we use when we detox on New Year's Day. We set those New Year's Resolutions to start the year differently so we can see a change this time. But about 20 percent of us will give up on our resolutions after only two weeks into the New Year. We also use this when we are using twenty-one days to get a beach body.

How many of us are actually *using* the exercise equipment that's taking up space in our basements, family rooms, or garages? You know, the stuff we bought during the COVID-19 pandemic so we wouldn't have to go to the gym to risk being exposed. It sounded like such a great idea at the time when we made the purchases. Now the excuses living in our headspace are preventing us from getting the most use out of it. We tell ourselves that we'll start walking on the treadmill after we buy new running shoes. After all, our feet hurt, and we need better shoes. How many times have we bought an outfit to work out in? The matching jacket, the top and the bottoms. Don't forget the headband and the sweat socks. I mean God forbid someone catches us in uncoordinated fitness gear. And, ladies, how many of us say we can't work out because we just got our hair done? This is a very real and ever-present issue with black women as Black hair care is notorious for getting in the way of our regular workouts, especially when it comes to swimming. We don't want to mess up our mane. I have experienced it personally and I have witnessed it time and time again how cute hair trumps fitness for the African American woman.

These are just a few reasons why we don't initiate change today. We've all done it. Tomorrow, we promise ourselves. We'll do it tomorrow. When all we really have is the gift of today. We need to make deposits into our wellness banks daily. Why? Because we hope to be able to make withdrawals later. If we're blessed to grow older, we'll need lots of reserve. I mean don't you want to spend time with your grandchildren? Or attend friends' retirement parties. Or attend your class reunion. Don't you want to take a cruise with your significant other? So, let's vow to quit making excuses, eliminate our mental barriers and initiate change today once and for all.

## IMPROVE YOUR ACCESS TO HEALTH CARE

As you pursue better health, there are recommended evaluations (examinations, lab work, and studies) depending on your age group that you should schedule. Whether you have health insurance, private or public, or you go to a free clinic, access to health screening is a necessity for disease prevention and screening. Knowing your numbers can make the difference between preventing illness versus treating them. What numbers am I referring to? Blood pressure, BMI, glycosylated hemoglobin, waist circumference, lipid panel to name just a few. Let's discuss blood pressure first.

## A. Blood Pressure

Almost half of all adults in the United States and 40 percent of African Americans as young as twenty have hypertension or high blood pressure. It's the condition whereby the pressure inside the arteries is elevated requiring the heart to work much harder to pump blood throughout the body. It may result from genetic predisposition. Or it may come from excess stress, smoking, poor diet, excess sodium intake, too much alcohol, or excess body weight. Hypertension may be asymptomatic in most cases. But may also cause symptoms of headaches and dizziness. It is a major risk factor for strokes, heart attacks and sudden death. Therefore, routine screening is advised from age twenty and beyond. If you are diagnosed with hypertension, I caution you not to ignore it. Understandable, you may want to tackle the diagnosis on your own, but I suggest partnering with your healthcare provider for a strategy to improve your numbers. Maybe this could include medications or lifestyle plan of diet and exercise. Get yourself a time frame and follow up regularly because the effects of untreated hypertension could be deadly.

## B. BMI

Body Mass Index (BMI) is a screening tool that was developed years ago to estimate the amount of fat on a person's body. It's calculated by measuring weight in kilograms divided by height in meters squared. BMI is a very controversial tool as it attempts to classify weight as underweight, normal, overweight, or obese, but it cannot quantify the distribution of fat on the body. Although there are limitations, BMI is an excellent starting point and predictor of risk of disease.

Normal BMI is less than 25. Overweight is 25 to 29.9 and Obesity is defined as 30 to 35 (class I) 35 to 39.9 (class II) and 40 and above (class III). Knowing your BMI is an excellent start to improving your weight or maintaining it. When I measure a patient's BMI, I also discuss the entire body composition to put into perspective how patient's BMI may affect their current state or the future of their metabolic health. I review body fat percentage and compare it graphically to others in the same age group. I also look at muscle mass and review norms. Hydration status is another parameter that I discuss as well as amount of visceral fat. These numbers together give me so much information as it relates to health. It allows me to develop a plan of action of improvement as well.

## C. Glycosylated Hemoglobin or HbA1c

HbA1c is a screening test for diabetes which measures the amount of glucose carried on the membrane of the red blood cells. It calculates the average blood glucose over the preceding 120 days, which is the lifespan of the red blood cell. A normal HbA1c is less than or equal to 5.6 mg/dl which equates to a blood sugar of 100. 5.7 -6.4 mg/

dl is borderline diabetes and equates to a blood sugar somewhere between 121-130. 6.5 or greater is classified as type 2 Diabetes and suggests blood glucose levels that are 140 mg/dl or greater.

Forty million people are diagnosed with type 2 diabetes each year in America. Diabetes screening should be done to rule out not only the presence of diabetes but prediabetes as well. Knowing this number empowers you to make wiser decisions about your body your nutrition and health. For instance, knowing that you are prediabetic allows you to choose a low carbohydrate diet, begin an exercise program and avoid or at least delay the diagnosis of diabetes, one of the leading causes of premature death in our country.

## D. Waist Circumference

The number of inches measured around our waists is called the circumference. We can all admit that a slender waist is perceived as sexier, more attractive, and desirable than a beer belly, muffin top, or spare tire. A six pack is most enviable, but it will not be easily identified underneath the layers of fat that comes from a poor diet. Knowing this number, is a gauge of how much body fat we have. How do we measure it? Take a tape measure and measure your waist just above the hip bones. A measurement for women greater than 35 inches and for men greater than 40 inches is viewed as unhealthy and has been associated with an increased risk of heart disease, diabetes, high blood pressure and high cholesterol. A large waist circumference suggests a larger than normal accumulation of fat around the viscera (the vital organs such as the liver, the intestines etc.) not the subcutaneous fat or fat beneath the skin. This fat is metabolically active which means it secretes hormones and chemicals that are inflammatory and increase the risks of all the aforementioned diseases. Additionally, excess visceral fat has also been linked to cancers and even Alzheimer disease. No amount of sit ups will eliminate belly fat. It can only be addressed by nutrition, calorie imbalance, and other lifestyle intervention such as lowering stress, getting sleep, and doing cardiovascular exercises.

## E. Lipid Panel

Lipid screening should be done on routine physicals to assess cholesterol levels which can determine our cardiovascular risks. Cholesterol which made by the liver is required to make hormones in the body and maintain the integrity of the membrane of our cells. Our bodies produce cholesterol naturally, but we also get it from our foods. A typical lipid panel includes **total cholesterol** which should ideally be equal to or less than 200mg/dl. **HDL or high-density lipoprotein** is the 'good cholesterol' and is responsible for removing excess cholesterol from the blood stream and carrying it to the liver where the body can either use it or excrete it. And **LDL or low-density lipoprotein** which is the "bad cholesterol" that increases our risks of heart attacks.

Normal HDL is greater than or equal to 60mg/dl. A high level of HDL has anti-inflammatory effects in the body and is linked to a lower risk of cardiac disease. The number of HDL may have a genetic link, but it also may be influenced by our nutrition and lifestyle choices.

Let's review the many ways to increase our HDL cholesterol.

A. Increase consumption of healthy fats, rich in omega 3 fatty acids such as olive oil, walnuts, and salmon.

B. Eat a diet low in simple sugars such as donuts, bread, Doritos, and cookies.

C. Exercise regularly. Studies show that high intensity work outs tend to raise HDL the most significantly.

D. Eat coconut oil. One study suggested that women who had a larger amount of abdominal fat but ate more coconut oil had reduced LDL to HDL ratio. More research is needed, but only two teaspoons of coconut oil per day may be impactful by lowering inflammation in the body by raising HDL levels.

E. Smoking cessation. Smoking suppresses the formation of good cholesterol and the function of HDL as well raising the risks of heart disease so just don't do it.

F.  Lose weight. How you lose weight may be questionable, but research shows that it increases HDL and is healthier for the body.

G.  Eat purple produce. These contain anthocyanins which fight inflammation and protect cells from free radicals and potentially raise HDL. The foods rich in anthocyanins are eggplant, red cabbage, blueberries, blackberries, and black raspberries.

Ideal LDL or low-density lipoprotein should be less than or equal to 100 mg/dl. Many factors can raise LDL including family history, smoking, high fat foods, obesity and leading a sedentary lifestyle. There are many things that we can do to lower LDL.

A.  Eat more protein from plant sources than animal sources. Yes, my vegan friends! Animal fat will increase LDL. And according to nutritionists, this means all animals, including chickens, fish, cows, pigs, and lamb.

B.  Exercise more. It lowers LDL and reduces fatty plagues in the arteries.

C.  Drink green tea. Studies show that it lowers LDL in overweight individuals or those with increased risk of heart disease.

D.  Eat nuts.

E.  Stress less.

F.  Eat more soluble fiber such as beans, apples, pears, and Brussels sprouts.

When all else fails, be open to the idea of medications, which may be lifesaving. The recommendations for cancer screening tests depend on your age and risk factors and should be discussed with your primary care doctor so that you can develop strategies for early detection, prevention, and treatment. This requires diligence. And there is no one more worth it than you so let's get on the books to get our checkups to empower ourselves today.

## SAY YES TO YOURSELF

A woman's nature is to be a caregiver. From the moment we see the angelic faces of a newborn, an incredible emotional connection ensues. We lovingly make sacrifices of love to raise our children. From infancy to adulthood, we nurture them to ensure that they become responsible well-adjusted members of society and can carry the torch of becoming parents of the next generation of children. Then we become caretakers to our aging parents helping them navigate their aging process. Helping them with their doctors' visits and activities of daily living. Sometimes our roles literally switch before our very eyes as we seem to become the parent and they become the child until they are no longer with us. Unsurprisingly, women are often the heart of the home managing everyone's schedules, preparing the meals, car-pooling, helping with homework, arranging doctors' visits, extracurricular activities, and to top it off, many of us work outside the home as well.

Many women have very demanding careers or jobs that require large amounts of time. It's no wonder we put ourselves last on our list of priorities. I mean with that kind of schedule, something's got to give. Right? But why is it usually us? Because we're overtaxed, overburdened, and over-committed. Does this mean we always have to say no to ourselves? We need to learn to say no more often to other things in order to say yes to ourselves. How can we delegate a little more and enlist a little more help? There is no shame in asking, requiring, or demanding help from our partners, neighbors, churches, social groups, or family members. Why not? Do we think less of ourselves if we must ask? I had this problem.

It took me years to admit that I silently suffered from the "I'll do it" syndrome. Maybe it's because I'm the oldest daughter or because I am just independently driven to get things done. But when it's to my detriment, it's foolish. Now I shout from the rooftop. HELP! 911! Stat! Throw a sister a lifeline. I don't have anything to prove. I want to preserve my health, my sanity, and my mind for things I want to do. If we're broken down, sick, or, heaven forbid, deceased, who's going to take care of it? Someone else that's who! I'm not suggesting that you neglect your responsibilities and obligations to your family or friends, but don't you at least deserve a little of that earnest concern? You are much more resourceful to your loved ones when you are your healthiest, happiest version of yourself. So, learn to say yes to yourself in small ways every day. Affirm that woman in the mirror and let her know that she is worthy of self-care and self-love and that her health and well-being deserve a bit more time, dedication, and commitment. Say it with me. "I deserve to show up for myself by taking care of my health needs. I will get rest, proper nourishment, and exercise for a strong, healthy body that will take care of me for the rest of my days."

## CHAPTER 2

# Examine Your Relationship with Food

## FUEL YOUR BODY

One thing I'm indifferent about is cars. It doesn't matter to me whether I drive a hatch-back, sedan, or SUV. I'm not a car-lover. I'm not a car aficionado. When my kids were younger, I drove a minivan that was so beat up that my friend Sheila taunted me about it relentlessly. The vehicle was so bad that I once while entering the hospital parking lot, attendant came to the gate and said, "This is the doctors lot ma'am, you can't park here." Another time I drove up to the front door of the hospital to *valet* my van and group of senior citizens tried to get in. Well, I upgraded my driving experience when that van finally broke down, and I was told by the salesman that I could only put premium gas in the car because it was a "luxury" vehicle and other gas would negatively impact the engine and potentially ruin the lifespan of the car. This same principle applies to our bodies which are fueled with a balanced combination of macronutrients to function properly. Our macros are foods that supply calories and consist of carbohydrates, fats, and proteins.

Carbohydrates are composed of sugar, starches, and fiber and are broken down into glucose into the bloodstream. Each gram of carbohydrate provides 4 kcals of energy. How quickly the body digests the carbs determine whether it's simple or complex. In general, the complex carbohydrates are the healthiest ones often referred to as the good carbs because they are rich in vitamins, minerals, water, and fiber. Get it? They're complex. They take longer to digest so they keep blood sugars stable without unnecessary spikes and keep us nice and fuller longer. These are our fruits, vegetables, beans, legumes, and whole grains. In contrast, simple carbohydrates, as I like to tell my patients, simply don't have much nutritional value at all. They taste good though. The quicker rise in blood sugar triggers an emotional response that makes us crave them more and more. I'm talking ice cream, milk chocolate, and red velvet cupcakes. If sweets aren't your thing, how about savory? Alfredo pasta, french fries, or fried chicken and waffles? Let's face it. We love to eat these foods, but they increase our risk of excess weight and type 2 diabetes.

Proteins are the building blocks of every human cell and are comprised of amino acids. There are twenty different amino acids that make up each protein molecule which are either essential (which comes from a food source) or nonessential (produced naturally by the body).

We get 4 kcals of energy from every gram of protein consumed. Proteins are derived from plants and animal sources. They build strong healthy hair, muscles, skin, and bones. Plant-based proteins come from foods like broccoli, Brussels sprouts, beans, nuts, and seeds. Animal-based proteins come from whey or dairy as well as from seafood, eggs, beef, and poultry. The National Academy of medicine recommends that we eat 0.8 mg per kg of body weight each day. Other sources recommend 1 mg per kg. After age forty, we begin losing roughly 1 to 3 percent of muscle per year. This is known as sarcopenia. The effect is a slowing metabolism and propensity for weight gain. We can combat this with consuming more protein each day and engaging in more muscle building exercise.

Dietary fat is an excellent source of energy that allows the body to absorb fat soluble vitamins which are vitamins A, D, E, and K. These vitamins are important for vision, bone health, immune function, and coagulation. Fat supplies a whopping 9 kcals per gram eaten. This means that we eat double the number of calories for every gram of fat we eat. There are good fats and bad fats. The bad ones may increase our low-density lipoprotein (LDL) cholesterol which is a major risk factor for heart disease. Red meat, processed meats (such as bacon and sausages), butter, and cheese are examples. An easy way to remember the difference between the two kinds of fat are that saturated fat (tend to be solid at room temperature) and unsaturated fat tends to liquid at room temperature).

The American Heart Association recommends limiting saturated fats to < 10% of your diet. This means that if you eat 2,000 calories a day, no more than 200 calories should come from saturated fats. Monitor your fat intake. Eat more fish than red meats more olive oils than butter. Limit processed meats and eat more fresh fruits and vegetables.

We can add value to our lives and not take away from them. Food can be performance enhancing or depleting as a fuel source. Fast foods, junk foods, and excessive alcohol consumption increase our risks illness including heart disease, diabetes, and cancer just to name a few. The Standard American diet is saturated with highly processed, fat-laden, and artificial ingredients that contribute to poor health. I recommend choosing a healthy combination of complex carbohydrates, protein, and fats rich in omega-3 fatty acids to maintain the best energy and improve our outcomes.

But just making the right food choices sometimes isn't enough to meet our goals. Let's talk about intermittent fasting as it pertains to eating a healthy diet because the management of our nutrition not only involves knowing what to eat but also when to eat it. Through my journey of working with my metabolic scores and managing my weight during menopause I have found intermittent fasting (IF) to be an absolute gamechanger to my existence. Everything I had learned about nutrition came into question when I learned about IF. Eating multiple times throughout the day. Breaking a morning fast early every day. Is this really the best way for everyone to eat? Or must your metabolic profile be considered. After all, no two people are alike and therefore one concept cannot apply to all people. I needed to seriously do more research on this topic.

## WHAT IS INTERMITTENT FASTING?

Intermittent fasting, also known as intermittent energy restriction, is the principle of voluntary periods of fasting in between periods of calorie consumption which has been studied as a way to reduce the risk of diet-related diseases. It has been shown to help with obesity, insulin resistance, hypertension, dyslipidemia (abnormal cholesterol panel), and inflammation. Although the US Institute on Aging said in 2018 that there was insufficient evidence to recommend it, the American Heart Association believes that it produces weight loss and lowers insulin resistance and cardiometabolic diseases.

Dr. James Fung, a Canadian nephrologist, is one of the world's leading experts and a staunch advocate of intermittent fasting. He commonly treats patients with type 2 diabetes and has written three best-selling books on the health topic. He recommends IF for many adults who are either struggling with their weight, have been diagnosed with type 2 diabetes or need to improve their health for other reasons. He does not recommend it for children, adolescents, or pregnant and breastfeeding women. With that said, let's discuss the types of intermittent fasting, and I will share which type I have incorporated which has been effective during my menopausal state. Again, let me clarify that this is not a diet. I am not a proponent of diets to lose weight. As an obesity specialist I am a proponent of a way of eating that one can incorporate and sustain life-long to assist in achieving or maintaining a healthy weight and prevent or reverse lifestyle diseases that we are plagued with in the USA. With that being said, let's dive into intermittent fasting.

There are generally six approaches to IF that have been described in the medical literature.

*Alternate Day Fasting*

The first approach is alternate day fasting. With this, one will either fast completely or eat one high-quality calorie meal of roughly 500 calories every other day. This meal must be rich in protein and therefore may include a large salad packed with meat, fish, or eggs. A small portion of added chickpeas or beans and pumpkin seeds would really add to the nutritional value of this meal. During this time, you may drink plenty of water or zero-calorie beverages such as black coffee or teas to remain hydrated and stave off hunger. This approach may be difficult to sustain long term and has been criticized as not the most efficient way to lose weight.

## 16:8 Method

The 16:8 method involves restricting eating for sixteen hours of every day and allowing yourself to eat a healthy diet within an eight-hour window. Within that time, you can eat two or three meals. Many people who don't like breakfast will typically eat this way. Those who really enjoy breakfast can consider having breakfast foods with your first meal no matter what time you break your fast. Here is another important point. For this to work effectively, the meals consumed must be healthy ones, not processed and junk foods. It defeats the purpose if you pig out during this eating window or make very poor food choices.

## 5:2 Diet

The third method is the 5:2 diet. This method of eating involves eating a sensible diet of healthy foods five days a week and on two days restricting your calories to approximately 500 to 600 calories. This style of eating was popularized by a journalist in Britain by the name of Michael Mosley. It's suggested that the total calories be split up between two smalls meals for the day and of course hydrating well will plenty water is recommended. This has been shown to be very effective in helping achieve weight loss. You may choose any two days you want to do this. Make it easy and sustainable and it will work.

## Eat Stop Eat Method

The next intermittent fasting method is called the eat stop eat method. This in my opinion may be the most challenging, but it involves fasting from breakfast one day to breakfast the next day. Or from lunch to lunch. Or from dinner to dinner. Basically, you fast so that you complete a full twenty-four hours of fasting. Eat stop eat may be done one to two days per week and again your regular meals must be simply healthy meals.

## The Warrior Diet

The fifth method of IF was made popular by Ori Hofmekler, a fitness expert, and is similar to the paleo diet. It is called the warrior diet. During the day, you are allowed to eat small amounts of fresh vegetables and fruits. At night, over a four-hour window, you eat one huge meal.

## Spontaneous Meal Skipping

The sixth and final method of intermittent fasting is called spontaneous meal skipping. I think is one fast that almost all do, whether it's on purpose or unintentional. The spontaneous meal skipping method is based on the principle that if you are not hungry or able to eat a healthy meal, just skip it altogether and allow yourself to resume your normal eating at the next meal.

All six of these methods of intermittent fasting are based on the premise of voluntary food restrictions based on timing of foods but assumes that the quality of foods chosen during feeding periods are healthy. If we don't purposely avoid junk foods, fast foods, and overly processed sugars, and fats, we will not see the changes we seek. For me, the goal is a slim waistline and maintaining an excellent body fat percentage for my AARP age group. Additionally, it's keeping normal blood pressure and fasting blood sugars. Every year that I don't require dialysis is a blessing and an absolute victory. Not being prescribed cholesterol lowering medications and requiring costly doctors' visits, procedures, and hospitalizations are a win. I have been using the 16:8 method, and I have personally noticed improvement in my blood pressures and blood sugars. When I say improvement, I mean I've gone from having borderline high elevations in my blood pressure during times of stress to totally stable. Also, like 80 million other adults in the U.S., I was tipping on the border of diabetes even though I was normal weight, exercising regularly, and eating sensibly. After incorporating 16:8, my blood sugars have improved substantially.

## FEED YOUR EMOTIONS

How many of us eat because we're stressed? Perhaps we've experienced the breakup of an important relationship. We might be facing an important deadline at work or maybe we're just plain old bored. This can trigger food cravings and the urge to overeat in effort to soothe our feelings. It becomes habitual just like drinking in excess or using illicit substances. What we really need is to address our psychological issues. What are we really feeling? If we're sad, let's create positive strategies to address it. Chocolate cake can't help us through it. What it does is stimulate the receptors in the brain that release dopamine. This neurotransmitter triggers a sense of reward which of course is temporary and most certainly addictive. The better we feel the more we want to continue to feel good. This cycle of eating to feel better can lead to overweight and obesity. Perhaps therapy is one way to address our life stressors. Certainly, prayer and meditation are positive ways to help us through difficult times. Family relationships and connection with friends may strengthen efforts to get through tough times. I have found self-help books and motivational literature as things I enjoy to assist me through tough times.

Stress eating may not be an issue for you. You may be the type of person who eats excessively at celebrations. When you're attending a bridal shower, time to get your grub on. When you attend a birthday bash for your best friend, time to chow down. At your niece's baby shower, get your eat on. Your wedding anniversary, time to feast again. It is such a blessing to have things and people to celebrate in life, but these are sometimes excuses to eat and drink uncontrollably. Now, you have to wear Spandex just so that when you overindulge you won't feel so uncomfortable. You eat and drink more than the people who are actually getting married, celebrating an anniversary, or giving birth. Is it really about the festivities and the fellowship, or has it now become about your excuse to eat your way into a frenzy? If you're watching your numbers on the scale get higher and higher or if your muffin top is spilling over your belt, you may need to reevaluate these habits. You absolutely should be able to attend festive events and enjoy yourself without jeopardizing your health or your waistline. But similarly, some of us eat to celebrate any and every special occasion.

Maybe you're a party girl and you look forward to happy hour cocktails. You enjoy a couple of drinks on the weekends at the local winery. Or you love your Wine Wednesdays. Alcohol use is associated with loss of inhibition. Moreover, drinking affects the part of the brain that monitors self-control. When we drink, we're more likely to consume foods high in sugar and fat. When we overdo it at times this gets us in big trouble with our weight. We must learn to address our feelings without food, attend celebrations without overindulging, and develop strategies to soothe and celebrate ourselves without ice cream, chocolate bars, potato chips, or french fries. Food is not meant to comfort us but give us energy to live our best lives.

## FRESH IS DEFINITELY BEST

Through my struggles with food, I've discovered that enjoying a healthy palate is an acquired taste. The standard American diet is composed mostly of processed foods, which are low in fiber and high in saturated fats. Simple sugars such as those found in breakfast cereals, potato chips, snack cakes, and soda are vastly increasing our risks of overweight and obesity. Although most ready-to-eat foods are very convenient, they're often packed with preservatives. Since the 1940s, antibiotics and growth hormones have routinely been given to farm animals to feed the masses of people. Does this affect our health in any way? According to the US Department of Agriculture, there is no evidence that antibiotics in foods are harmful to people. But that doesn't change the fact that the typical Western diet has been linked to cardiovascular disease, diabetes, and cancers. According to an article published in the *Center for Science and Public Interest* called "Why Good Nutrition is Important," almost 700,000 deaths per year are attributed to an unhealthy diet. Moreover, obesity rates have doubled in US adults, tripled in children, and quadrupled in adolescents. That's just crazy right? How can kids not outlive their parents? This subject is very controversial and has two contrasting views. One thought is that due to diseases related to poor eating habits and lifestyle our children may not outlive their parents. Another opinion is that they will indeed outlive us but will unfortunately suffer the burden of comorbidities such as diabetes, strokes, and obstructive sleep apnea that decrease their quality of life and increase the costs of healthcare.

Let's face it, our taste buds have been super saturated with additives and artificial ingredients. We are so used to added fat, added salt, and added sugar that we've developed a preference for it. Even finicky toddlers recognize McDonald's golden arches early in their food journey and start to request some fries and chicken nuggets from the back seats of mom's minivan. Unsurprisingly, eating whole food in is its natural state rarely increases disease risks. How many raw foodists, vegans, and vegetarians do you see in the cardiology clinic in line for a heart transplant? Very few indeed. The original fast food grows on trees, on vines, and from the ground. Eating food in its natural state has been thought to decrease inflammation. Whereas heating and processing foods are thought to destroy many nutrients and enzymes in them. Unprocessed and unpasteurized foods are thought to increase energy, help in weight loss, and improve vitality.

Let's challenge ourselves to rethink our choices. Incorporate more of a whole food diet rich in fruits, vegetables, nuts, and seeds to fight signs of aging.

Eating nuts will give your skin a beautiful glow. Green leafy vegetables keep the skin firm and smooth and enhances circulation. The boost in antioxidants will promote strong and shiny hair. Blueberries contain anthocyanin which prevents collagen loss. There's an array of delicious foods to try!

## FOOD IS NEITHER FRIEND NOR FOE. IT'S JUST FOOD

What is your relationship with food? What does food mean to you? Is it based on family traditions or social trends? Do you have a love hate relationship with food? Are your eating habits influenced by your childhood? Did your parents influence how you clean your plate? Were you ever made to feel ashamed about your eating, the amounts of food you eat, or your choice of snacks? Sometimes we carry this emotional baggage into adulthood. And we develop an unhealthy relationship with food. Does eating healthy food make you feel good about yourself whereas indulging in a slice of cheesecake causes you to ruminate all weekend about how bad you ate? These extremes in thoughts about food aren't healthy. See that's just it. Food is not good or bad, it's just food. We often judge ourselves too harshly when it comes to food. We think all good or all bad when we should think of food in terms of more healthy or less healthy.

An unhealthy relationship with food can lead to both eating disorders and excess weight. Anorexia nervosa involves the act of withholding calories to the point of approaching near starvation to maintain a perceived healthy weight. Women are more likely than men to suffer from anorexia. Adolescents are more at risk for this disorder. This may result in electrolyte abnormalities, heart conditions or even death. Bulimia nervosa is the act of binge eating then inducing vomiting or taking laxatives, diuretics, or other stimulants to lose weight. Bulimia can cause tooth decay, depression, and abnormalities with electrolytes. Other eating disorders are binge eating disorder and night eating syndrome. Binge eating disorder is characterized by episodes of recurrent binge eating and associated by negative psychological problems. Those with night eating syndrome tend to eat most of their calories at night. They tend to binge on high-calorie foods and eat in shame. They're more likely to suffer from guilt and depression and being overweight is very common is this class of eating disorder. Finally, Body Dysmorphic Disorder is a mental illness where there is a perceived obsession with one's appearance. One is obsessed with flaws in her body that no one else seems to see.

In my opinion, it's better to take an 80/20 approach to eating your macronutrients (fats, protein, and carbohydrates). Decide to eat sensibly most of the time and save your less healthy options for special occasions. Even if you eat less prudently on holidays, your birthday, an anniversary, and a couple of baby showers for the year, you still have many more opportunities to eat better. Excess weight doesn't usually result from the now and then splurge. It results from the poor choices we make on a daily basis.

Too much fast food. Sodas every day. Nightly desserts and cocktails all contribute to unwanted pounds. If you can change your thinking about food and put it in its proper place, you can achieve a balanced mind and body.

Remember that food is not meant to be your friend or your lover or a long lost relative. It's just meant to nourish your body.

## GET OFF THE DIET ROLLERCOASTER

What's your latest diet this time? Whose detox are you trying now? Is it Beyonce's Master Cleanse where Queen Bey lost twenty pounds in just two weeks to get ready for her role in the movie *Dreamgirls*? In this diet you avoid eating solid foods entirely, only to replace it with a drink of water, cayenne pepper, pure maple syrup and fresh-squeezed lemon juice. Or are you doing the JJ Smith Ten-Day Green Smoothie Detox, which claims to help you lose up to fifteen pounds in only ten days? What supplements are you taking to lose weight? Vitamins and minerals are important to aid in overall health to supplement your im-perfect nutrition, but just to help with weight loss? Not going to happen. Some nutritionists believe that extreme dieting puts us at risk for vitamin deficiencies. They lack protein and adequate amounts of fiber and are impossible to sustain. I suggest ascribing to a way of eating and stick-ing to it is the best way to manage your weight with the least amount of effort. Whether you eat a Mediterranean diet, low-carbohydrate diet, or paleo diet, just stick to it. During the COVID-19 pandemic, I resolved to eating at home. I refused to eat any junk food or fast foods. I took all my meals and snacks to work with me and under no circumstances did I eat out. I concentrated more on a whole food, pescatarian diet and with very little effort and lost weight during the pandemic.

As stated previously, losing weight has not always been my focus. My effort to avoid the diagnosis of type 2 diabetes has been my most important objective. I've chosen a nutrition plan that supports disease prevention and allows me to maintain a healthy amount of body fat. My plan just happens to be a low-carbohydrate pescatarian lifestyle which allow me to liberally consume fresh vegetables, low glycemic fruits, whole grains, and wild-caught fish. Does that mean I don't eat guacamole? Chips and salsa? Or my favorite red velvet cake sometimes? No, it doesn't. I just try not to overindulge.

Restrictive dieting is a concept of all or nothing eating that is usually unsustainable and leads to rebound weight gain. Decreasing calorie intake causes a shift in hunger regulating hormones and a slowing of metabolism which attempt to preserve the body and prevent starvation. After dieting ends, and regular eating resumes, a slower metabolism combined with an increase in calories over time leads to weight regain and the disappointment of another attempt to lose weight and maintain it. Experts believe that 95 percent of all diets eventually fail.

As a weight loss expert, I can tell you that even though the weight loss market suffered a 21 percent decline in value during the COVID-19 pandemic, the epidemic of obesity is not going anywhere. The weight loss industry is expected to grow 2.6 percent every year through 2023 simply because people are expected to continue to grow. We are seeing younger and younger people struggle with weight issues. Diet companies are acquiring other companies. Multi-level marketing companies are getting a piece of the action with promoting and selling various products. Weight-loss franchises are popping up and weight-loss surgeries are becoming more common. Prescription drugs are great options for many people, but the insurance industry does not want to provide enough coverage for all those who could truly benefit. I'm a firm believer that people need a solution-based approach to their weight problems. Choose a way of eating that gives you the desired benefits and stick to it. Scientists say that your way of eating should be personalized, and not trendy.

## CHAPTER 3

# Embrace Exercise as Medicine

## SET YOUR ALARM EVERY DAY

When you want something bad enough, I mean really want it, you make a lot of sacrifices to get it. You pencil it in. You add it to your calendar. You block out the things, circumstances, and even the people who stand in the way of it. It takes the forefront of your attention. After menopause, my designated workout time had to be restructured. But I still had to pencil it in. Exercise must be prioritized. Making time for it is something that any woman with a spouse, children, or a job or responsibilities of any kind must figure out. The challenges don't go away. Your game strategy just gets better. Set your alarm daily to get up a few minutes earlier each day to work out. Or at your lunchtime or at your kid's volleyball practice. It doesn't have to be hours of exercise. Just minutes. The American Heart Association recommends thirty minutes of moderately vigorous exercise five days a week to keep our hearts healthy and strong. That's approximately 150 minutes each week. But it doesn't have to be five sessions. The time can be broken up however you see fit. Ten minutes here, ten minutes there, it all adds up. Set the alarm on your smart phone to remind you to move more throughout the day. Use one of the dozens and dozens of apps on your phone to pencil in fitness. Once per hour set your alarm to get up and move.

Sitting all day will age you. Your bones. Your joints. Your muscles. And your skin. Try calisthenics, some stretching, or jump rope. One of my favorite impromptu workouts is Seven, the Apple app that allows its users to do seven minutes of high-intensity interval training (HIIT). Let's compare two types of exercise that I find beneficial in helping women to age gracefully: low-intensity steady state exercise (LISS) vs. high-intensity interval training (HIIT). Some experts suggest that a healthy combination of the two types of exercises is beneficial with 20 percent of our workouts consisting of HIIT and the rest consisting of LISS.

Low-intensity steady state exercises include walking, swimming, yoga, cycling, and hiking. These workouts help reduce pain, burn fat, and improve posture and cardiovascular fitness.

According to an article entitled "Seven Benefits of High-Intensity Interval Training" published in *Healthline*, HIIT has seven major health benefits. The first way is that it allows us to get the maximum amount of health benefits in the minimal amount of time. The second is that it boosts your metabolism for hours after each episode. Number three is that HIIT can greatly reduce body fat and your waist circumference. The fourth benefit is that even though weightlifting is the gold standard for muscle building, HIIT can increase muscle gain. Reason number five is that HIIT, compared to endurance sports, can improve oxygen consumption. The sixth reason is that it reduces heart rate and lowers blood pressure. And the seventh reason is HIIT reduces blood sugar and can improve insulin resistance even more than traditional exercise. The best part of it is that it requires no equipment, no weights, just you, boo.

## FIND YOUR COMMUNITY OF SUPPORT

The greatest asset to my fitness lifestyle was discovering several communities which supported me in my fitness journey. I was the quintessential bookworm all through elementary school. Although I was very interested in learning gymnastics, I came from a very modest upbringing and my parents couldn't afford for me to take lessons. I learned to do basic tumbling and even became a cheerleader but that was it. In high school I didn't participate in any sports activities. My high school was an all-girl school, and we didn't have many intramural sports. We didn't even have a swimming pool. By the time I went to college, I took a few aerobics classes and even explored dance classes to my extreme enjoyment and my family's surprise. But it wasn't until I attended medical school, when I realized the benefits of exercise and the importance of maintaining good health, that I began exercising more regularly.

Because my athletic husband could not support my amateur efforts and often left me in the dust when I tried my luck at running, I sought out other support. My cohorts from the YMCA were my first group of supporters. I met a friendly group of people at the Y who regularly took aerobics classes together. We started doing more exercises before and after classes and struggled through ab challenges together to enhance our fitness. It was so motivating to enjoy the encouragement and support of others on a similar quest to get in shape.

Next, a colleague at work told me about a unique multi-sport fitness group composed of women of color called Team Dream. This group was started by a Triathlete named Derek Milligan, who was incredibly passionate about the sport of triathlons. He is a skilled swimming instructor and loved teaching a technique of swimming which is a training method used by swimmers to improve performance by practicing gliding effortlessly through the water as opposed to exerting excess energy and fighting through the water. This is an ideal method of swimming for the triathlete who needs to preserve her energy for the biking and running legs of the triathlete race. This amazing training led to me participating in and completing two sprint level triathlons. And it was the beginning of my love of an active lifestyle. My next beloved group, called Women Run the World, was started by an amazing woman named Jae Rockwell. She started this fitness community to help women in their quest to walking, running, biking, lifting or whatever they enjoyed. The group enjoys meet ups and check ins to encourage and motivate fitness. This led to me completing over twenty completed races, from marathon relays to 5k races to half marathons.

And finally, Black Girls Run, a national organization, led me to participate in multiple training runs, several obstacle-course races and one Ragnar Relay. It also led to many forever friendships that filled endless hours on the running pavement. I've been enormously inspired to try new things and push myself way out of my comfort zones due to my community and I am forever grateful to these groups

## MAKE HEALTHY DEPOSITS

Chances are that when we were younger, we weren't exactly thinking about metabolic scores or BMIs. We didn't give hypertension or osteoarthritis a second thought. These were our grandmothers' issues not ours. Now that I'm a GG, my focus is a lot different. Every time I go to the doctor for a checkup and receive a good report is like going to the bank and withdrawing a million dollars. It's invaluable. I believe as the saying goes, that our health is truly our wealth because without it, we can't achieve true freedom. The liberty to pursue things that make us happy and fill us with purpose. Every race I've participated in, I could almost predict how well or how poorly I'd do based on how much training effort and how much time I put in to prepare for it. When I put more effort into my workouts, I saw the results. When I didn't put forth the sacrifices required to train whether it was due to my busy work schedule, family obligations, or my laziness I felt more of a struggle. Usually, the sacrifices required me to give something up in order to achieve my higher objective which was to have fun completing my races and seeing what my body could accomplish.

My next investment into my health was good food. Now I don't think this investment required a lot of money, but it did require a little bit of forethought and planning. Planning meals around training required me to be able to shop, prepare, and cook the foods that I knew would provide the sustenance I needed for better energy and performance. I'd rather eat junk food and fast food sometimes, but it often left me feeling sluggish. Having a couple of drinks is fun when you are at your favorite restaurant, but it almost always makes me tired and dehydrated the next day which is not motivating at all to get out of bed and to the gym early. And all those protein shakes, big salads, and chicken breasts for dinner can sometime seem monotonous, especially on pizza night.

The investment of gym equipment, exercise videos, personal trainers, fitness coaches, and the visits to the gym, all the days and nights on the pavement placing one foot in front of the other would culminate in the thrill of completing a race.

Still need more motivation? Here are five reasons why we should invest in our health and make these deposits:

Reason Number 1: Good health can reduce health costs. How many of us want to spend all our retirement pension or social security on health care expenses, medications, and hospital bills?

Reason Number 2: We get to spend more time with those we love. We'd rather spend our golden years creating memories and not being a burden to our family.

Reason Number 3: Healthy lifestyles can prevent diseases. Research confirms this and as Hippocrates says we should let food be our medicine and medicine be our food.

Reason Number 4: We're more productive when we're healthy. At work at home and in society.

Reason Number 5: Being sick can make us unhappy and miserable. Suffering and living less than our best lives is not what any of us desire. Living with regret and remorse is a dreadful thing to experience let alone to watch. I can remember witnessing my paternal grandfather in an ICU bed in the hospital after suffering a stroke, crying, unable to use any words to communicate with the family. I saw his only son, my father weep for his dad. I wondered if he had regret over some of his life choices. He appeared to know what he wanted to say to us but could not express in words what was on his heart and that made him weep. As a young adult I didn't quite understand everything that was going on but remember the sadness and pain on the face of my father who prayed for a miracle that his dad would recover. Sadly, he did not and soon passed away. My grandfather spent a lifetime being a cigarette smoker and having hypertension, I'd wondered if he wished that his life was different.

As someone who comes from a family with a strong history of diabetes, hypertension, cancer, heart disease and obesity, I strive to avoid these diagnoses every single day. But to make regular withdrawals, I focus on making frequent deposits. My deposits include stress-reducing activities, healthy food choices, and a variety of movement. Every time I do yoga instead of lying around—deposit. Every time I favor walking to my office instead of driving—deposit. Every time I lift weights instead of playing games on my cell phone—deposit. Every time I cycle instead of scrolling on social media—deposit. Be willing to make the necessary deposits every day to have a hefty withdrawal. It's worth it!

## USE DISCIPLINE AND REPETITION

We live in a microwave society—in a right here, right now type of world. We don't want to work for much. We want to look a certain way without putting in any effort when it comes to our appearance. But permanent change usually requires some effort. Of course, there are a few exceptions to the rule. Some women seem to be able to do what they want, eat what they want, and never move a muscle yet still they have a body enviable to most. But that's not my story. I really put in the work. I used to wonder why it seemed like things were so hard for me. Why couldn't things just come easy? Honestly, I don't think I would appreciate it if things came so easy. Have you heard the saying that Rome was not built in a day? Well neither is a banging body. You got to put in that work, girl. Don't get discouraged when you don't see immediate results because change rarely comes over night. No matter how much you want it to. There are a lot of work outs, spin classes, walks/runs, Zumba classes, cross fits, Pilates classes, P90X sessions, HIIT, and Peloton rides between you and the body of your dreams. A whole lot. I always advise my weight loss patients to choose an activity that they enjoy so that they don't mind doing it very often.

The key to staying disciplined is to vary your activities to keep things interesting. Be willing to try new things and think outside the box to avoid boredom. Challenge yourself to keep an open mind. Can a disciplined lifestyle be fun? It absolutely can. Moreover, it is an incredible feeling to look and feel amazing as a result of all your hard work. To feel energetic and enjoy increased strength is empowering. Varying your activities and recipe swapping prevents boredom. Finding fulfillment in your purpose takes precedence. I personally enjoy participating in challenges to keep things exciting. I thrive in goal-setting and healthy competition. Find out what keeps you on task and go for it.

The difference between success and failure in achieving your goals is not giving up on yourself. So many times, I have started and stopped a routine. Many days, work got in the way, or I was derailed by obligations or responsibilities. That's life. You can't always change it, but you can control your response to how you handle certain obstacles in your life. I say all the time that I sometimes feel like a professional hurdle jumper. It feels like the barriers of unexpected happenings in life, have trained me to jump higher and higher. Sometimes they're unexpected and oftentimes they're unpredictable. Occasionally they're close together and other times they're far apart. Sometimes I clear the hurdles with ease and other times I don't, causing me to fall flat on my face. Or on my knees and elbows. I wear those battle scars of life's hurdles with pride. Some of those scars are superficial and some are deep. But none of them are deadly. If I live to die another day, then it's a testament that it isn't over yet. God has more for me to do.

The most incredible sports example I was able to witness while participating in a triathlon was watching a blind triathlete completing the race as well. She swam a half mile across a man-made lake with the assistance of swim angels at her side. They encouraged her and guided her through the water until she surfaced on the other side of the lake's beach to the thrill of observers of the race. Then she was led to a bicycle built for two where she preceded to bike 13 miles up and down a hilly countryside of the course until she was ready for the final leg of the race. Finally, this amazing athlete ran 3.1 miles alongside a companion who again assisted her in staying on the guided trail of the race event. This extraordinarily brave soul completed the Danskin Women's Triathlon without even the gift of sight. How brave and determined she was to even attempt such a daunting feat. This was a tremendous example of fortitude, discipline, and determination which resulted ultimately in success! I knew then that if she could do it, I could too. There are no limits on what we are capable of, only the limits of the mind and will. That year I completed my first triathlon. Watching that visually challenged participant influenced me to train harder determined to return the following year to perform a personal record.

## HONOR YOUR TEMPLE

1 Corinthians 6:19-20 (ESV) says "Or do you not know that your body is a temple of the Holy Spirit within you, whom you have from God? You are not your own, for you were bought with a price. So glorify God in your body."

Amen! This resonates with my spirit. And fills me with great encouragement every time I read it. I'd like to think that the human body is a work of art. And what an amazing work of art the human body is indeed! How can I glorify God with my body? Let's me count the ways. I can think of a few ways. Fill it with positivity. Give it food that provides it with good energy. Move it and enjoy the strength it gives me to praise God with it. Allow it to serve me well as I serve others which is a privilege.

3 John 1:2 (KJV) says "Beloved, I wish above all things that thou mayest prosper and be in good health, even as thy soul prospereth." God created the most incredible thing when he created us. Our bodies are the most intricate, unduplicatable, beautiful combination of systems ever created. How everything works together, and although studied greatly, most people can't even begin to understand it. How dare we defile, abuse, neglect, or take this amazing gift for granted? It should be revered. We should honor it by taking care of it. It's meant to move and thrive not to sit and fester. We can't avoid the process of aging but we sure can slow it down by investing in frequent movement. The goal is to get it to be able to take care of you and not require the assistance of others, especially the healthcare system.

I spent many of my younger years trying to change who I was, instead of embracing who God made me. I felt I was too short, or I didn't like the sound of my own voice.

I worried that my breasts were too large, or I didn't like the way I looked. I'll never forget when I was an intern, my patients would embarrass me by asking to see the doctor when I would enter their room. Do you remember Doogie Howser M.D.? It was a television drama about a teenage prodigy who was challenged with being both a young-faced adolescent and a doctor at the same time. I was mortified that my patients mistook me for the medical student more times than I can remember. Back then, I silently wished that I looked older so that I could avoid these awkward encounters with my patients. After all, I had worked incredibly hard to earn my doctorate degree and trained endless nights to achieve the respect that I thought I deserved. These embarrassing situations occurred for many years as I was carded well into my thirties. And even now, I am often mistaken for being many years younger.

Now that I'm older, I am thrilled to be mistaken for a younger woman. Are you kidding me? Why in the world would I want to look older? God has blessed me with a youthful appearance that I believe comes from the spirit. It stems from my outlook and how I view the world. Proverbs 17:22 (ESV) says, "A joyful heart is good medicine, but a broken spirit dries up the bones."

I try to see the good in people and not the bad. I have an optimistic view of the world and am filled with childlike hope that things will always be better. This is a gift from God, I honor it. I embrace my youthful spirit. Every quirk and imperfection make me who I am. And I am special to my heavenly Father. My temple was created to honor God and I accept the charge each day with gratitude.

## CHAPTER 4

# Get Your Beauty Rest

## SHUT IT DOWN, SIS

Ever since I can remember, I've gone to bed relatively early. My aunt used to say that I played so hard during the day as a child that at night I simply passed out at night. My childhood best friend, Andrea, used to say she didn't know how in the world I got through medical school, when I'd often be out like a light every night before the news was on television. I'm embarrassed to say that nine o'clock has been my bedtime since I can remember. In fact, I don't know how in the world I pulled all-night study sessions in college, medical school, and residency. Or staying awake for forty-eight-hours for that matter. And to add fuel to the fire, I chose obstetrics and gynecology as a primary career, which almost always requires working overnight. How in the world did I do it? When I'm not working, I always go to bed early. My body prepares for the opportunity to rest. Sleep is the place where the body restores itself. Our cells replenish themselves and the body rejuvenates during periods of sleep which is divided into four stages. And each stage has a purpose.

The four categories of sleep are awake, light sleep, deep sleep, and rapid eye movement (REM). As our bodies progress through the stages of sleep our bodies transition through various processes that affect breathing, temperature, muscle, and memory.

Studies show that not getting enough sleep and interrupted cycles of sleep contribute to metabolic disorders that lead to chronic health conditions, including weight gain, and obesity. It's thought that sleep deprivation contributes to dysregulation of the hormones that control both hunger and fullness signals in the body. Those who don't get enough sleep tend to have greater hunger signals promoting the tendency to not only eat more but to choose fatty and sugar laden foods. Poor sleep is associated with oxidative stress and glucose intolerance which increases the risk of diabetes. People who are sleep deprived also have decreased energy and are less likely to exercise, which is essential to our overall health and maintaining a healthy weight. I can't begin to tell you how many workouts I missed after being up all night on call. All the runs I missed and training sessions I couldn't attend. After many years I realized that my career choice sadly was contributing to my poor health habits and to my own insulin resistance (prediabetes). Another scary thing I have experienced in my life are night terrors, known as parasomnia. The difference between a night terror and a nightmare is that the night terror occurs in stage three of sleep as opposed to REM sleep. It may be associated with screaming, sleepwalking, or profuse sweating. I can't tell you the number of times I have jumped from my bed screaming as though Michael Meyers from Halloween was chasing me. I have felt dreadfully sorry for my husband who has witnessed this. And although night terrors may have many causes, sleep deprivation is thought to be one of them.

Fortunately, I have gotten back to practicing medicine in a way that allows me to sleep most nights. I believe that it is helping me keep it all together, reducing stress, my waistline, and those frightening episodes.

## CIRCADIAN RHYTHMS

The effect of light and dark on the body in a twenty-four-hour period is referred to as the circadian rhythm. This guides our bodies and lets us know when to sleep and when to be awake. During the day, our master clock or brain sends signals to the brain that keeps us alert and active. At night, the brain produces melatonin which promotes sleep and helps us stay sleep throughout the night. Circadian rhythm assists with metabolism by regulating blood sugar and cholesterol. It also helps with our mental health and may be associated with potential for depression and even diseases like dementia. Circadian Rhythms are linked to the immune system and cancer fighting cell repair.

Everyone's need for sleep is different. Some people are early risers and others are night owls. I personally need much more sleep to feel refreshed and effective throughout the day. In my obesity assessments, I examine patients sleep habits and assess how they either enhance or block weight loss. What I consistently find is that those who are sleep deprived either due to work schedules or menopause struggle to lose the weight they want to lose. Especially my doctors and nurses and my swing-swift workers. Studies reveal that those who work during the night or swing shifts are more likely to have issues with weight suggesting that the lack of sleeping during certain hours of the day may have effects on our hormones that contribute to weight maintenance.

I'm a perfect example of a person who struggled with metabolic health. My circadian rhythm had malfunctioned. With chronic sleep deprivation and being awake hours and sometimes days on end, I developed insulin resistance or prediabetes and borderline Hypertension despite working out and eating a reasonably healthy diet and maintaining a normal weight. How could I lecture others about this very thing when I was living proof of what not to do?

## HORMONES AND WEIGHT GAIN

Weight is a most complicated phenomenon. The Obesity Medicine Association defines obesity as a chronic relapsing, multi-factorial, neurobehavioral disease, where an increase in body fat promotes adipose tissue dysfunction and abnormal fat mass physical forces resulting in adverse metabolic, biochemical, and psychosocial health consequences. Whoa, now that was a mouthful. It's influenced by a multitude of factors including nutrition, sleep, movement, genetics, hormones, and behaviors. When we're sleep deprived, our adrenal gland produces more cortisol, which is our flight or fight hormone, that is made is response to more stress inside the body. If we make more cortisol this also triggers the release of ghrelin, the major hormone produced in the stomach that increases hunger signals. But not just hunger, I'm talking major cravings. We want donuts, soda, and cheeseburgers. It also inhibits leptin. Leptin is a hormone which is produced by the adipocyte or fat cell that regulates energy by telling the body when we're full and have had enough to eat. This chronic imbalance of hormones most certainly leads to weight gain.

Moreover, excess cortisol or stress hormone also increases the production of insulin which is manufactured by the beta cells of the pancreas that increase the risk of insulin resistance and diabetes. Insulin is the hormone that regulates the metabolism of glucose by promoting the absorption of glucose from the blood into the liver, fat, and muscles. It's a major contributor to the storage of fat or excess weight. The tug of war between the neurotransmitters of the brain and the hormones in the body give credence to the fact that losing weight is not simply just about eating less and exercising more. Unfortunately, it's way more complicated than that.

## SLEEPLESS NIGHTS AND FATIGUE

Working nights is a sure way to drain your energy, but you don't have to work graveyard shift to have sleep issues. Sleepless nights cause fatigue, and as a result, your body lacks the stamina to take on various tasks. Exercise requires energy. If you're tired, you don't feel like going to the gym, working out, or taking a Zumba class. You just feel like going to sleep or laying around surfing the web. You may feel tired and tend to spend time doing unproductive things like watching TV. Even if you do make it to your work out, you're more likely to be less effective than if you were well rested.

Add to this the onset of menopause which may be characterized by waking up multiple times throughout the night due to hot flashes and night sweats. The presence of menopausal symptoms and lack of adequate sleep can result in sheer exhaustion during the day. This time where women will naturally experience a decline in reproductive hormones which typically occurs between age forty and fifty-something is defined as menopause. For me, this was age fifty-one, the average age of menopause in American women. But some women experience menopause after the surgical removal of the ovaries referred to as an oophorec-tomy. The change in a women's hormone levels can lead to absolute drain of energy and symptoms of chronic fatigue. Some women experience every side effect of menopause and others experience none. How do you best beat these symptoms? Rest and meditation are often ways to assist with low mood. Regular exercise is a great way to release endorphins and improve quality of sleep. Limit caffeine intake and alcohol use which may interrupt sleep cycles and cause nighttime awakening.

Fatigue is also common in those with obstructive sleep apnea (OSA). OSA is a sleep-related breathing dis-order characterized by complete or partial blocking of air passages while lying down. It is seen more often in those with obesity, chronic nasal congestion, men, and older adults. Those with this condition may have reduced or al-most absent breathing episodes which reduces oxygen to the brain. A bed partner may notice symptoms of loud snoring, choking or even gasping for air. The next day one can experience day-time sleepiness or fatigue. A CPAP machine which expands the collapsed upper airway can improve nasal breathing reducing the symptoms of OSA ultimately reducing the associated risks of hypertension, arrhythmias, and heart problems. Losing weight may completely reverse the effects of OSA. I suggest a sleep study to make the diagnosis and talk with your primary care provider if you have any questions about it.

## TURN OFF YOUR DEVICES

How many hours of the day do you spend on your cell phone? How about your iPad? Your laptop? What about your television? I admit that I spend entirely too much time on my devices. Posting for social media. Reading my emails. Basically, I use my phone as a computer to manage my business. It honestly drains me. Personally, I'd rather not being doing it at all. I miss the simple time when I felt free to be alone with my thoughts and daydream. When I was growing up in the 1970s, television programming went off promptly at 11:00 p.m. The Star-Spangled Banner would play, and all television programming would be discontinued until the next morning. There was no cable television.

Cell phones were nonexistent. If you wanted to have a conversation, you'd have to go into the kitchen and use the phone that was attached to the wall. This ensured shorter conversations because you'd have to stand up until you got off the phone. If you had an emergency and needed to contact someone and weren't at home, you would have to find a pay phone, insert 20 cents, and make a phone call. Am I dating myself? There were no personal computers. We used typewriters and encyclopedias. My kids can't conceive of such a time! With the initiation of modern technology, cable TV and twenty-four-hour programming it is common for people to watch television into the wee hours of the morning, surf the web nonstop, and play

PlayStation for hours on end. We are exhausted as a society and just aren't getting enough sleep. There is direct correlation between poor sleep habits and increasing BMI in the U.S.A.

Up to 35 percent of adults don't get an adequate amount of sleep. According to a National Poll of the National Sleep Foundation, 95 percent of people use some sort of electronic device within an hour of going to sleep. And to make matters worse, 75 percent of us use these devices in our bedroom. Because these devices stimulate our brains it makes it harder for us to fall asleep and the blue light emitted from our smart phones and other devices disrupt the natural production of melatonin made by the brain to facilitate sleep. For this reason, it's recommended that we make the bedroom a device-free zone and get back to better sleep.

## CHAPTER 5

# Make Yourself a Priority

## YOU CAN'T POUR FROM AN EMPTY CUP

Whenever I'm not taking enough time for own wellness, I feel terrible and notice how it impacts my mood. I don't feel my best. My sense of empowerment is diminished. I feel less optimistic. Pessimistic even. As a wife, I may be less than excited about taking care of my husband's needs. In turn this affects my ability to be the best wife I can be. How can I make my husband happy when I'm less than joyous? It is difficult at best.

As a physician, I assist my patients in their wellness efforts. I help them achieve their desired goals of losing weight and maintaining good health. This requires my intentional listening and strategy to assist them in their efforts. My clients pay me for and depend on my expertise. However, it's difficult for me to be solution driven when I'm distracted or overtaxed. I make time for conferences and continued education. My professional development and enhancement is a lifelong journey and needs regular attention. I need time away to reassess where I see myself both in the medical space and as an entrepreneur. Moreover, I must constantly learn and grow as a professional.

My greatest contribution to the world is being the mother of three uniquely wonderful individuals: Edward, Courtney, and Caitlyn. They have taught me so much about myself, the world and how I see myself in it which has humbled me in ways I can't begin to explain. I have needed to tap into and surround myself with supportive family, neighbors, and friends to raise them successfully from birth into adulthood. Now, as they've grown into young adults, I realize the importance of always staying centered even more. I can't help them in their personal endeavors if I don't stay grounded in my own foundation which is God. My physical, spiritual, emotional health and well-being must be prioritized. Taking care of myself means making time to focus on my own personal growth and pursuit of purpose. It wasn't until I was approaching my fiftieth birthday that I thought I had discovered and was living in my unique purpose. The GPS of life takes many twists and turns. There are times when you find yourself in a place where you did not expect to be with people who you'd rather not be in your space. This has happened to me many times before. This is the perfect time for introspection, recentering and then beginning the task of decluttering.

I've always been a goal-setter. In school although I wasn't always the smartest person in the class, I was certainly the one who tried the hardest. In fact, I was voted the most likely to succeed in my eighth-grade class. I thrive on living from goal to goal whether I'm training for a race, renovating my house, or deciding to start a business. This requires that I pencil myself in and can take care of my mind, body, and spirit. Any upset in the apple cart, results in an unhappy me and that never works. Take the time and prioritize yourself. Fill your cup every day and don't apologize for it. You are worth the effort and the dedication.

## YOU DESERVE BETTER, GIRLFRIEND

What I continuously see in women who are struggling with weight, is that they somehow have talked themselves out of believing that they truly deserve the transformation that they seek. As a result, they engage in self-sabotaging behaviors. The closer someone gets to their goals, the more they will inadvertently get in the way of their own success. They may abandon their healthy eating or their regular exercise routines. Why in the world would they do that you may ask? The fear of change. Sometimes we have associated who we are with what others have identified us to be. Instead, we must empower ourselves to accept change and improvement. This explains why even after losing a great deal of weight, people don't seem to notice how different they look.

I can recall times in my life when things were so incredibly amazing, I would think "This is too good to be true" even after I intently prayed for it. Even though I had all the qualifications for it. God is able to do exceedingly abundantly above all we could ever ask or think. How dare I be surprised. I am His daughter. I must get comfortable sitting at the table He has prepared for me before my enemies. We must get comfortable attracting great things, people, and situations into our lives and know that we deserve them. Why not you? Why not now? Aren't you worth it? You must believe that you are. Accept your blessings. Live in your purpose. You deserve it, sis, and you are certainly worth it!

## LOVE WHO YOU SEE IN THE MIRROR

Self-love is the greatest gift that you can give yourself. It's not your partner, not your children but yourself, second only to God. Unfortunately, many of us have experienced life situations which have been a blow to our self-esteem. Whether we've been abused in a relationship, divorced, suffered the loss of a family member, or lost a job or career. God thought enough to you to create you as a singularly unique individual. Even if you're a twin and share your genetic makeup with another person your body houses its own individual mind and soul.

We must learn to love what we see in the mirror and not what we wish we saw. Sure, we all have something that we'd like to change about ourselves. Perhaps we'd like our thighs to be thicker or our stomachs to be flatter. If that's your case, work on it. But in the meantime, don't sell yourself short. Never use negative words when describing yourself. Stay positive and embrace who you are not who you'd rather be.

As we practice more self-love, try to let go of thoughts of perfectionism, which turns out is harmful to us. Perfectionism has been linked to adverse health effects and studies show that perfectionists are at greater risk for both mental and physical illnesses, including irritable bowel syndrome, fibromyalgia, depression and eating disorders. Silence your inner critic and release all forms of negative thoughts. You'll be happier in the end.

*Psychology Today* says that self-love involves four aspects. Each important in growing to love ourselves unconditionally. They are self-awareness, self-worth, self-esteem, and self-care.

Self-awareness means being aware of how your thoughts affect your own emotions and how they in turn cause you to act. Being self-aware involves being able to process these emotions effectively.

Self-worth is the belief that we have in ourselves. It is something that we just have. It is not earned or determined by outside influences. Rooted in the belief that we are valuable. We must learn to value who we are despite society's standards or cultural standards. Women have a harder time I believe than men with this so we should practice affirmations or seek counseling support or even self-help groups when necessary. Whatever it takes to be the best version of ourselves, we should strive to achieve.

Self-esteem is the idea that because we have worth, we are comfortable in being who we are. There is no need to justify our existence. Self-care is all the acts we do to keep ourselves healthy. It can be as simple as bathing or brushing our teeth to eating a balanced diet and enjoying our favorite hobbies.

## AVOID THE SUPERWOMAN SYNDROME

How many women do you know have been socialized to think that they need to be everything to everybody? Superwoman Syndrome, a term coined in 1984, is typically seen in women who take on multiple roles in her life which might even be detrimental to her own physical, mental, and emotional wellbeing. Women are socialized from the time we're little girls to take care of the family. We buy our daughters American Girl dolls, teach them to have tea parties, and play school where we encourage them to be the teachers not the principals and the school superintendents. We stock their toy kitchens with pot, pans, dishware, and pretend food to prepare them to be little cooks. Then, we expect our daughters to excel in college and become judges and doctors or lawyers right before they get married and have children. All the while society expects them to look like supermodels so they can keep their husbands sexually entertained and interested.

After our daughters' get married and raise children of their own, we then expect our daughters to take care of us. Honestly, we don't hold our sons to the same standard. Why in the world do we do this? I don't really know. This perpetuates an unrealistic expectation that women must live above normal expectations. According to Dr. Tasneem Bhatia's book, *Superwoman Rx*, there are five types of superwomen. The first is the *Boss Lady*, known for her intelligence and wit, but unrealistic demands can eventually increase the risks of her own health and happiness. The next type of superwoman is the *Savvy Chick*. She is more artistic. The third is *Earth Mama*, who is very caring and compassionate and often puts her needs last. Fourth is the *Nightingale*, who is very motivated by a sense of service and selflessness. You recognize her traits in many of your sorority sisters. Lastly, there is *Gypsy Girl*, who is very creative and imaginative. All these women may be prone to physical and emotional conditions such as anxiety, weight gain, insomnia, reflux, and constipation. Do you see yourself in these women?

This doesn't just happen in American culture; it happens in many others as well. It poses the risk of self-neglect, depression, anxiety disorders and even substance abuse. I see the effect of this in those struggling with overweight and obesity. There are greater risks of emotional eating and eating disorders including binge eating disorders.

The need to be all things to all people is a trait of the Superwoman Syndrome. Saying yes to others before we say yes to ourselves repeatedly can quickly lead to burn out, depression, and anxiety. Give yourself permission to take off your cape and send it to the dry cleaners every once and a while. While it's there, enjoy being normal every now and then like the rest of us mere mortals.

## CHAPTER 6

# Genetics vs. Environment (Work with What You Got)

## DO WHAT YOU CAN AND LET GOD DO THE REST

I often share the story of my family's horrible health history. My dad had a triple coronary bypass by the age of forty-nine. He suffered from type 2 diabetes, chronic hypertension, and became an amputee. He developed kidney failure and had to have dialysis to sustain his life. At the end of his battle, he suffered a stroke and had a fatal heart attack while undergoing dialysis treatment. When I got the call that my father had been rushed to the hospital after he collapsed in dialysis, my heart sank. I lived only three minutes away from the center to the south of me and three minutes to the hospital to the west. And when the emergency room clerk sat me and my husband in a private room for what seemed like an hour while we waited for the doctor to come update us on his condition, I instinctively knew that he was gone. My father coded and could not be revived after a battle with kidney failure due to complications from diabetes.

It was heartbreaking to watch my father go from being a healthy, happy-go-lucky guy who loved listening to music and singing to an amputee with failing vision that frequently talked about what he wished his life could have been. This was heart breaking for me to see someone I cherished practically deteriorate before my very eyes and suffer a premature death based on lifestyle diseases. Could his fate have ended differently had he been educated on the importance of eating better, exercise, behavior change, and weight loss? I think so. Every day I teach people how to make lifestyle choices which change their metabolic profiles. I've had diabetics go into remission. I've seen hypertensive patients become normotensive and discontinue their blood pressure medications. And how about avoiding the need for statins or cholesterol-lowing medications just by eating right? With all the debate about medication side effects being able to get healthier just by eating better, it's such a rewarding thing. In fact, it's a very common result that I see every day in my practice.

Obesity doctors agree that weight is a very complex issue. The debate of nature (genetic predisposition) versus nurture (environmental influence) has long existed. But by just changing your perspective and embracing one's willingness to change, I believe lives can be saved. Lifestyle medicine focuses on educating and motivating patients by changing personal habits and behaviors around the use of whole food, physical activity, restorative sleep, stress management, avoidance of risky behaviors and positive social connection. It promotes changing your lifestyle to combat your genetics.

Research shows that when there are certain brain receptors present in rats, it caused the rat to eat up to 130 percent more carbohydrates than others suggesting a biological link to eating behaviors. But human choices are also affected by our culture, the media, and social norms. In essence there is an interplay of genetics vs environment in the determination of our health and it's up to us to do our part.

## MY MAMA'S DAUGHTER

My mother was genuinely one of the most kind-hearted, altruistic people I have ever met. She was beautiful inside and even more lovely on the outside. and unbeknownst to me, she was a math whiz, a Sudoku puzzle expert, and amazing critical thinker. She, like many women, was a victim of childhood emotional trauma. She became a teenage mother and married early. The stressors of a failing marriage wore on her and she sought comfort in food and began to eat to soothe her emotions. I watched her exhibit symptoms of emotional eating and depression which led to serious health challenges resulting in obesity, type 2 diabetes, and eventually leiomyosarcoma (cancer of the uterus), which resulted in an untimely death. We daughters watch our mothers. Their habits and tendencies. And sometimes we tend to model them.

My mother often said to me that she believed her life could have been different if only she had only been educated about some things. If my mother had only told me things, I would have listened to her. I just didn't know any better and she did not teach me. This resonated with me and influenced me to take a different approach in mentoring my daughters; what I taught them and how I raised them.

According to an article published in the *American Journal of Preventive Medicine* called "Behavior Matters," behavioral interventions can effectively be used to prevent disease, improve management of existing disease, increase quality of life, and reduce healthcare costs. Behaviors are learned not inherited. Because of my background in psychology and medicine, I was able to identify that I needed to choose more positive ways to relieve some of life's more stressful situations. I was able to sincerely sympathize with my mom's life experiences. I am so grateful that she poured into me and influenced my decisions to make different life choices and explore positive outlets to stress. I chose to use exercise as an outlet to my stress and to try to avoid using food as a source of comfort or escape from life's stressful moments.

## YOUR DAUGHTERS ARE WATCHING YOU

As I mentioned previously, I was an observer, an admirer, and a witness to my mom's life. And because I knew my daughters were also watching their mother, I believe that I should demonstrate the behaviors that I suggested they too should follow. I tried to live by example because kids usually do what you do not just what you say do. It's important to set a good example for those who look up to you. Take them with you to your golf lessons. Play tennis with them. Invest in a family membership to the local YMCA or community center so that every time they watch you, they'll establish exercise habits as well.

Now that I'm older I realize that my daughters needed to see my naked emotions. My fears and insecurities. They needed to see how I deal with disappointments and struggles. I needed to unmask my vulnerabilities so that they could see that even doctors have fights with their husbands or may become estranged from their close friends or even cry sometimes in the basement after their mom dies. And that's okay. Being true to your real self is freeing. It eliminates the need for pretentiousness or the need to put on airs. It's acceptable to not have it all together or to need therapy. We need to look in the mirror and be content with our imperfections.

How do we accept our imperfections and love ourselves anyway? Don Dulin says in his article published on the website Unfinished Success that we must first make peace with our journey. Each of our life journeys are different. We're never at the same place at the same time. We should accept where we are and move on and that's perfectly fine. Understand that learning from mistakes is of the greatest benefit when we don't repeat them. Perfection is an impossible standard. You can always be thinner, fitter. Don't chase perfection because it has been referred to as a dead-end street. Find peace wherever you are. The final thought about imperfections is that negative emotions are a normal part of our human experience, so we allow ourselves to move through all the sad times, angriness, frustration etc. to pursue our happy place.

## YOUR EFFORTS ARE EFFECTIVE

You can change your outcome! You can push for better. You can absolutely overcome obstacles. I am not suggesting that your limitations and difficulty are non-existent. However, they do not define you or control your future. You are capable. You have the ability to be greater than your difficulties. Stay true to your goals and don't become a statistic or victim of your circumstances. Decide to win and then put in the work at all costs.

The fact that I am fifty-five years old at the time of this writing and have delayed the diagnosis of all the lifestyle illness of my parents and grandparents is a tremendous blessing. By the time my parents and grandparents were my age, they were spending a ton of time in their doctors' offices getting prescriptions, at the hospitals having expensive tests and procedures. They simply weren't educated by their practitioners on the benefits of lifestyle medicine or behavioral health habits. They were not given directives on how to lose weight and gain health. Nutritional counseling should be a part of every preventive health care visit. Doctors should not just instruct you to lose weight without instructing you how to do it. What type of foods are best for your health conditions? What's the difference between a calorie and carbohydrate anyway? How can you successfully incorporate more exercise in your life to lower your risks or at least improve your chances of aging more zealously and reduce chance of injury? Promote smoking cessation and incorporate support and accountability? People really do want to know that people care and that they can consult you when they need help.

I'd like to think that maybe my parents might have made different choices with the right education and guidance from a qualified physician who believed in lifestyle medicine and prided in herself on enlightening patients about the importance of disease prevention. Perhaps they may have lived longer or at least had a better-quality life. This is a testament that with God and strategic behavior change we can avoid many of the pitfalls that plague the American healthcare system.

## CHAPTER 7

# Build on Healthy Habits

## START SOMEWHERE

Start anywhere. An article published in *Medscape* in May of 2018 entitled "Adopting 5 Healthy Habits in Midlife Could Add 10 Years of Life" revealed that changing five simple habits during the ages forty-five to fifty-five may increase our lifespans by an entire decade. These are definitely worth mentioning.

Number 1: Never smoke. Don't puff. Don't vape. None of it. Not a cigarette, cigar, pipe, or other. Just let it go. Don't become a slave to tobacco, nicotine, and all the hazardous chemicals that are placed in tobacco products.

Number 2: Keep your weight within a healthy range. Defined as a BMI between 18.5 and to 24.9 kg/m2. I'm not going to get into the debate on how your family is big boned or that your culture carries weight differently. Or that BMI is a biased way to measure one's health. This is what the research shows.

Number 3: Exercise daily by doing thirty minutes or more of moderately vigorous activity. You choose the exercise. Move your body well and often.

Number 4: Eat a high-quality diet. What might that be, you ask? Of course, quality is relative but I'm certain that junk foods, processed foods, and fast foods aren't included in this.

Number 5: Limit alcohol consumption. Up to one glass per day for women and two glasses per day for men.

Getting started is the absolute hardest part of developing new habits. Eliminating old ones seems almost impossible at times. Preparing your mind to accept change is difficult because we feel so comfortable with the familiar. Nobody likes to change because it invokes a sense of uncertainty. We are generally creatures of habit. Old habits are very comfortable like an old pair of boyfriend jeans. Our activities of daily living are habitual. We shop at the same stores because when we go to a new store, we don't know where to find things. We buy similar foods because we tend to prepare the same meals over and over and over again. Even the way we prepare foods are learned perhaps from childhood. Whether we cook or eat out all the time. Small changes add up and the benefits are enumerable. Broiling meats instead of deep frying them is a better option. Decreasing the number of packaged dessert snacks such as Oreo cookies or Twinkies for fresh fruits. Substituting sodas or sweet teas for regular or sparkling water. Adding salads or vegetables to your lunch instead of potato chips. Taking the stairs instead of the elevator or enjoying a fifteen-minute walk each day.

## FOCUS ON ONE DAY AT A TIME

Yesterday is past. Tomorrow is not promised. But today is a great opportunity to really make an impact. Divide your day into thirds: morning, afternoon, and evening. Then divide it further into hours, minutes, and even seconds to maximize your opportunities to be more effective. When you realize that one hour is comprised of 3,600 seconds it seems more impactful that you can devote that entire time meal prepping, meditating, or exercising. Organization is the key to being more effective and optimizing your time. Cut out all your time-wasting activity. Who cares what celebrities are wearing? We all know that the Real House-wives aren't actually housewives. And as for social media, it's just a means to an end, as far as I'm concerned. There are only so many TikTok videos and memes on social media we can consume every day. We must get into the business of managing our time better to take better care of ourselves which requires a bit more time and a lot more attention. It's a challenge that I experience myself even to this very day. Each day has twenty-four hours. We are all given the same amount of time. What we fill it with varies. Just make sure that you are responsible for your own.

## FORGIVE AND FORGET

There are things I wish I'd done when I was twenty-three that I didn't do. There are places I'd wish I'd gone, opportunities never realized, and a boat load of mistakes made.

But that time has passed. It's behind me. I must learn to forgive myself and graciously move on. I can't change the past so why linger there. It's counterintuitive to today's plans. Why do we women allow ourselves to be held hostage to our past? Some of us can't soar in the present because we can't heal from yesterday. It's like a scab that we keep picking. No wonder we can't build something new. We're obsessed with the do-overs of yesterday. News flash! It can't happen. Start building today on what you have today. Now say along with me, "I forgive myself" and I'm worth another chance. Now doesn't that make you feel hopeful?

Likewise, I've held on to a few grudges and had some unsettled disputes in my lifetime. In essence, I allowed the past to rob me of a peaceful present. I held on to unforgiveness. Whether I did not forgive people or situations in which I thought I was wronged by someone else. Either way I've wasted way too much time and energy on unforgiveness. For this reason, I am truly sorry. I apologize to my younger self for wasting too much time stuck on past mistakes that I couldn't focus or didn't put in the effort to work on my future. Give yourself a break and get to the business of moving on. Don't be idle and unproductive. You can't get time back. So quit trying.

## MAKE IT YOUR LIFESTYLE

Get used to it, girl. This is your new normal. Embrace your healthy habits. I often say that unless you're planning on getting younger, you'll need to resolve to make change permanent. You'll need to plan on initiating these new habits and then build on them. Our metabolisms don't get faster as we age, they get slower. Aging is a bitch, but what's the alternative? We all know what the answer to that is. And we are not trying to talk about it.

When it comes to making lifestyle changes, consistency is key. Being consistent in our efforts will pay off in dividends. Do you have fat clothes in your closet? You know the one you wear because you can't fit in your usual clothes. You've got your pre-pregnancy jeans, your before-you-got-married dresses, and your before-I-went-to-law-school suits, and they're all a different size. That is so frustrating. I'll never forget that after I had my first child, my husband gathered all my blue jeans and gave them away to his sister without asking me. When I angrily asked him why he would take it upon himself to give away my clothes he replied that since I couldn't fit them, he thought I didn't want them. Well, my intention was to get back into my wardrobe, not buy a larger one. My jeans were a gauge for me to see how well my plan for losing pregnancy weight was working.

Our weight is going to fluctuate throughout the lifecycle. But our habits bring us back to balance and wellness. I did get back into my jeans, by the way. And a second time and a third time after that. And now that I'm menopausal and fighting the menopausal belly the same principle applies. I continue my health routine, so I don't need "fat clothes" in my closet.

# CHAPTER 8

# Embrace Your Most Authentic Self

## LAUGH OUT LOUD EVERY DAY

My husband, Edward, and I share a private joke where I often declare that I'm sure that I married a third grader because he hasn't grown up yet. The reason is because when he and I first met, we were eight years old and in the third grade. Back then I thought that he was the absolute silliest boy I had ever met. Loud. Obnoxious. I couldn't tolerate being around him, because I thought he was too playful and way too immature. You know girls are so much more mature than boys. Forty plus years, three children, one grandchild, and many gray hairs later, being able to laugh and play and have fun together has kept us extremely light-hearted and given us a sort of joie de vivre that a lot of relationships envy.

It is said that laughter is the absolute best medicine because it releases endorphins from the pituitary gland in the brain which act as feel-good hormones and act as pain relievers. It forms a sense of togetherness and is downright contagious. Laughter stimulates serotonin release from the GI tract which acts as an antidepressant. And finally laughing has an anti-inflammatory effect that protects the blood vessels and the heart.

If I didn't have a giddy approach to situations, there are many times where I might have allowed life's stressors to overwhelm me. I'm learning not to be too serious about certain things. I need to learn how to let my hair down hypothetically. Ed reminds me to color outside the lines sometimes and encourages me to laugh at myself. Life is too short to be so serious all the time so why not add humor in every possible situation. Talk about the crazy situations! We have overcome some serious obstacles in our lives, but God reminds us of how he's in charge of it all. Dark days are always brightened by the dawn of another day. I coauthored a book called *As the Wind Blows, Volume 2*, where I account my trials through medical school while my husband battled addiction. I have a belly laugh every time Edward tells me that he is going to write a book to tell his side of the story, which he says is the real truth. If you can't laugh at your past, what can you laugh at?

I honestly think that child-like laughter keeps us young and hopeful. Without allowing ourselves to be goofballs sometimes, we might have seriously slipped into some ruts that were impossible to escape.

## SCHEDULE FREQUENT DANCE BREAKS

I love dancing. It invigorates me and puts me in such a happy place. My endorphins soar to great music, and it takes me to an amazingly delightful place. I used to wait for special occasions, a wedding, a birthday, or an event to bust a move. Then I finally realized that I am the life of the party. My happiness isn't determined by anyone else. It begins and ends with me. I enjoy having a good time. Laughter and fun add value to my day. Dancing makes me smile or maybe it just makes others laugh at me. Either way, somebody's laughing so that's a good thing. On any given day, you may find me cutting a rug in my kitchen to my favorite music. This for me represents freedom and the opportunity to take control of my feelings, my emotions, and my happiness. It allows me to be uniquely me. To be uninhibited and free and have my own kind of fun and burn a few extra calories as well. My husband and kids think I'm hilarious, and honestly, I'm happy to oblige them.

I'd like to take some dance lessons in this next season of my life. I'm talking ballroom dancing, salsa, and Chicago Style Stepping. I'm hoping that my life partner will join me in this adventure. And what a way for us to stay in shape together, meet interesting people and have fun all at the same time. Dancing helps to develop muscles, tone the body, and improve posture. It promotes balance, coordination, and flexibility. And hopefully, it will prevent me from falling and breaking a hip.

## LIVE IN THE MOMENT

Do you live in the moment? Or do you plan all things well in advance? I used to have such a difficult time with planning around my work schedule that I wouldn't plan anything at all. I didn't plan to take my birthdays off or holidays with my family or special anniversaries or even events surrounding my children's school activities. It causes me anguish to tell you that my first-born still remembers that I missed his kindergarten graduation party at school when he was five years old. He recalls the balloons and the laughter and all the fun of the celebration, but he will forever remember his mother's absence.

Like countless times before and then after that, I was working. I was a young doctor dedicated to my patients and my career, but I was not nurturing the relationships into which I was purposed to pour. I am not proud of that, and I have apologized numerous times to my son. There have been many apologies. Heck, it's a wonder that I'm still married to the same man for so many years.

Unfortunately, I have seen doctors lose their lives suddenly and unexpectantly in the peak of their careers one too many times throughout the years which helped me to gain a new perspective on how I wanted to live the rest of my life. I decided to prioritize more time with my loved ones and if the opportunity arises to do something un-usual or out of the ordinary—go for it! I want to see my grandchildren's Christmas plays and attend the dance re-citals. Birthdays are blessings that I don't want to miss out on anymore, so I am ready willing and able to enjoy the day-by-day experiences with those I love.

## TAKE A CHANCE ON YOURSELF

One of my favorite quotes is "She believed she could, so she did!" I love it because it epitomizes my view on how a woman should live her life. And my mother specifically gave me the confidence to try new things. She made me feel loved unconditionally and often verbalized that good or bad, succeed or fail, her love and support would always be waiting for me when I needed it.

I vividly recall sitting on my porch as a child day-dreaming about how I wanted my life to be when I grew up. And what I envisioned was like nothing like what I was accustomed to. My parents were a loving working-class couple who supported my endeavors. And because they knew I had big dreams they sacrificed to send me to pri-vate school so I could explore the possibility of a greater life. They gave me the courage to be the first of many. I was the first to go to college. The first to attend medical school. The first to own my own business and to become a published an author.

I gained the courage to try new things. Boldly and unafraid. I became determined to be the first doctor in my family. Despite all odds, I applied and was admitted to my first choice, Northwestern University. Then continued my medical education at the University of Illinois at Chicago, the largest medical college in the country and my dreams of becoming a doctor came true. I went on to receive not just one board certification but two. And now, I am the first female entrepreneur of my family as well.

Between every success I've had, there were many struggles. Honestly, I've failed at more things than I care to mention. But I refuse to believe that I can't accomplish what I set my mind to do. I have happily discovered that one is never too old to take a chance on oneself! Of course, there are things that I haven't done that I hope to do. The sky is truly the limit.

## SURROUND YOURSELF WITH OTHER UNICORNS

You know you're not like other people. You see the world entirely differently. You stand out from the crowd. If you're bored with the status quo, and usually color outside of the lines, you're probably an outlier. There's nothing wrong with your unique outlook. It took me fifty years to finally find my way off the beaten path. I so enjoy being around people who dream of amazing things. People who envision the world differently. I joined a travel club just to be around other unicorns. I've joined professional organizations to fraternize with other unicorns. I'm absolutely drawn to people who think outside the box. People who don't want ordinary things. Why? Because my whole life I have colored inside the lines and done everything I was taught to do. To do what? Fit in. But baby, age fifty hit me like a lightning bolt, and I decided that I had better do all the things I want to do before I leave this earth. Life is too short and too precious to just fit in and make do.

Now COVID-19 has put a huge monkey wrench in my life plans, but, hey, what can you really expect from a pandemic? I'm just excited to be here! I have seen too many negatively impacted by this global pandemic. Family, friends, patients, colleagues, and church members alike. I appreciate the blessing I see in things that I didn't see before. I'm grateful for every single moment and it's as if a dark veil has been lifted from my eyes allowing me to take in all the colors. The sea of gray and dull has been parted by flickering, bursts of rose gold and I love it.

# CHAPTER 9

# The Secret to Senescence

## LOSE YOUR LIMITATIONS

One of the secrets to aging well is releasing the thoughts that age limits us. The changes to our bodies are inevitable but the process of preservation begins in our minds. Why can't we learn new things? Why can't we go back to school and perhaps enroll in college and obtain advanced degrees. According to the Guinness Book of world records, the oldest college graduate is Shigemi Hirata of Japan who was ninety-six years old when he graduated from the Kyoto University of Art and Design.

Seasoned seniors are amazing contributors to the world and must not be overlooked. Ethel Davey from England supports her community by volunteering in a local thrift store every week. She started at the ripe age of seventy-eight and has not missed a shift in more than twenty-one years. She shares her talents with the world by giving her time. What cause are you committed to? Is there a place in the world that you feel you can still contribute to make a positive impact?

One of my personal favorites and an inspiration to my own pursuit of fitness is Ernestine Sheppard. She is, at the time of this writing, the oldest female body builder in the world. What impresses me the most about her is that she began her journey at age fifty-six when she decided to change her life for the better. Ms. Ernestine and her sister began working out to improve the appearance of their bodies and what happened was that a fitness revolution was started.

But I don't have to go far to be inspired by seniors who are challenging the norm and beating the odds of aging well. I have the pleasure of knowing two amazing women who call themselves the Seasoned Sole Sistas. Their names are Dancin' Mary and L.A. aka Hollywood. Dancin' Mary's nickname comes from her passion of being a line dance instructor. She is a married retired employee of the State of Illinois and supports other women in their running journeys. L.A. aka Hollywood is the firecracker of the pair and always the life of the party. She's a retired Chicago police officer, all of one hundred pounds, and is always down for whatever when it comes to a challenge, especially fitness. These two ladies are such an inspiration to healthy aging that I call them the Joint Chiefs of Fitness. They are spending their retirement running ultramarathons, jumping double Dutch rope, and doing whatever they damn well please.

Making such a commitment at such late age is by no means an easy task. The dedication it takes to not only get in shape after menopause but to do the type of workouts to get such an amazing transformation is no joke.

If we put our minds to it, we can do anything. My mom always said that although the body is aging, the mind feels as young as you allow it. Have you ever wanted to take on a new hobby? Learn a new language? Visit exciting new places? The sky is the limit for you. There's no reason you can't do it just because you're of a certain age. So, let's get to it.

## HAVE THE COURAGE TO CONTINUE

What do you do when your children have all grown up and embarked on the beginning of their lives, from finishing college to starting their new careers, completing graduate school, falling in love, getting married, and starting their own families? This is bliss. Isn't this everything you've ever wanted? From the time you decided to become a parent and an adult and began planning out your life. You've created the legacy that you intended. Where do you go now? What do you do with your time and energy?

It's not over for you. It's time to develop the courage to continue this adventure called your life. Heck it's time for you to reinvent yourself. Bask in new freedoms and possibilities that you've always dreamed of. It's exciting to pick up things you delayed years ago before starting a career and raising a family. This is called the second half. Part two. After the intermission. Things really get good now. It's finally time to put yourself first again. How does this sound for you? Exciting huh? Now you need to continue your journey of being everything God has called you to be. Now is the time to renew your commitment to yourself. What promises did you make to yourself as a little girl? Did you keep them all or did you leave some by the wayside? Now's your time to get the courage to get started again.

It's time to get started on keeping some of those promises you made to yourself. What have you vowed to complete? A bachelor's degree? A 5k race? How about becoming a homeowner? An author? What hobbies do you enjoy that you've been putting on hold? Gardening? Learning a new language? Traveling? Don't give up on your dreams.

## THE VALUE OF YOUR VILLAGE

As we age, we can experience many losses. We may lose a bit of our flexibility, our strength, or even our hearing. I swear that one day I literally woke up and my knees decided that we were not doing deep squats anymore. Our vision may change, and a very common part of aging is that we become hyperopic or farsighted, a condition where our ability to focus on nearby objects is impaired and we start needing reading glasses or bifocals. Because we don't see as well as we used to, we now need readers to focus on the small print of a newspaper, magazine or on the computer screen. Or in my case, my ability to cut the suture in surgery suddenly became challenging unless I looked over the top of my glasses. I had been nearsighted since the sixth grade. Now I am both near and farsighted. Damn! We may sadly experience the loss of a of parent(s), friends, or even a beloved spouse. These are crucial times where we need support. Friendship. Love. Maintaining close contact with our church groups, neighbors, family, and friends is an invaluable source of support and strength during our aging process.

I lost an elderly neighbor during an unexpected scorching hot autumn day in Chicago. She lived alone and suffered a heat stroke after failing to open her windows in 100-degree weather. Nobody checked on her. I failed to check on her. I should have done a wellness check on her and maybe I could have changed her outcome. I felt like shit when this happened. And every time I think about it, I feel sad. I know now that aging well involves having a healthy amount of social and physical interactions in your life. Studies suggest that depression and overall risk of mortality may be lower in seniors who get heathy amounts of emotional and social support.

## THE POWER OF POSSIBILITIES

I am super excited about what lies ahead. I am enjoying life to the fullest, whether I'm alone or in the presence of others. I love meeting new people and challenging myself to do new things. What I fear most is the thought of missing out on life and all its possibilities. I sacrificed a lot of my youth to study medicine while my friends were hanging out at the club, partying, and living their best lives. I was mostly knee-deep in the books. Attending endless study sessions and tutorials. One day sort of blended into the next day sometimes with endless deadlines, exams, and papers to write. From marriage to motherhood to the wonderful experience of becoming a grandmother, life has taught me many lessons. I'm continuing a journey of self-discovery and fulfillment. I've served and have enjoyed being a servant leader. I don't regret the decisions of my youth. I now know that everything I've gone through was to prepare me for where I am today. But now I want to travel the world with my forever boyfriend, Edward. Ideally, I'd like to start on the west coast and work my way to the east. Then we'd head overseas to explore different cultures and cuisines. We've always been either too busy or didn't have enough money. Our lives have been busy raising and educating our children building a home and working in our careers but now it's our turn to seize the moments. The thought of not having to set our alarms in the morning or answer our phones and text messages absolutely thrills me. I absolutely love the idea of being free and uninhibited in this next phase of life. Maya Angelou, the esteemed poet, said that life is not measured by the number of breaths we take but by the ones that take our breath away. As I see it, aging healthfully allows us to really appreciate the gift of life and enjoy the sun rises and the evening breezes.

So, what's in store for you in this season? Whatever you darn well please! It's time to make a bucket list of all the things you've ever dreamed of. Visualize all the things you want to do. The places you'd like to visit and hobbies you'd like to try. Haven't you always wanted to foster kittens? Or take tennis lessons? It doesn't matter. Whatever floats your boat. Turn your just do it into a just did it! In fact, expand your "been there done that" references and place a check mark by all the items on your completed list.

Healthy aging allows us to do all the things we desire to do in a way that we desire to do it. I am up for the charge. Are you?

# Conclusion

This year will mark the beginning of my fifty-sixth rotation around the sun and I can't believe how quickly the time has passed. Recently, I reflected with a colleague on how alive I feel and how excited I am to embrace this new season of my life. I'm becoming more open-minded and finally learning to think outside the box. I've developed a reasonable amount of confidence and security in who I am and want to live boldly. Bravely. Unapologetically. Gracefully. What's it going to take for you? Intention. It's going to take you being able to prioritize your wellness—mind, body, and spirit. Pause to allow yourself to live intentionally and purposely. Explore your uniquely adventurous journey and remain open to the possibilities.

Lower your risks and envelop a new body along with your new mindset. With it you can go anywhere you please. Set the standard then be the example you're looking for. Be the influencer of your own life. The star of your own story. Your happy ending is entirely up to you. How thrilling it must be to narrate the happy ending of your life.

Stand in solidarity with those who like you are in search of greater things. Be steadfast in your decision and don't turn back. Pause and take in all the excitement of what's in store ahead of you and not just what's behind. You won't regret it! Follow the roadmap and complete the steps to a healthier you. Be the baddest bitch in the room. She's definitely not perfect, but she allows herself to be perfectly secure in who she is and where she's going. If that's you than you are ready to join a movement of mid-life mavens who aren't afraid to be who they were born to be.

# References

Center for Science in the Public Interest, Why Good Nutrition is Important, March 21, 2016

Medscape, Adopting 5 Healthy Habits in Midlife Could Add 10 Years of Life, Marlene Busko, May 10, 2018

Medical News Today, Why Self-Love is Important and How to Cultivate It, Susan Sandolu, March 23, 2018

4 Ways to Accept Imperfection in Your Life, Don Dulin, December 2015

American Journal of Preventive Medicine, Behavior Matters, Edwin B. Fisher, PhD, Marian L. Fitzgibbon, PhD, and Judith K. Ockene, PhD

Healthline, How to Fight Sarcopenia (Muscle Loss Due to Aging), Matthew Thorpe MD, PhD, May 25, 2017

Cleveland Clinic, Women's Health, Menopause Weight Gain: Is It Inevitable? November 3, 2020

## About the Author

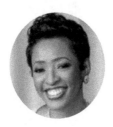

Dr. Goldwyn B. Foggie, a.k.a. Dr. Goldie, is a respected physician of twenty-five years, double board certified on the fields of OB/GYN and obesity medicine. She's a passionate advocate for women's health, especially the wellness of mid-life women experiencing the changes menopause brings about.

Dr. Goldie is the chief executive officer and founder of Illinois Wellness and Weight Loss Centers in Chicago, Illinois, where she has helped hundreds of clients transform their lives through weight loss and weight management. She is also the creator of Fit By Design, a community of women who prioritize themselves through fitness and self-care.

As a health and wellness expert, she enjoys speaking at churches, corporations, colleges, and conventions. She is also the author of the *Fit By Design Journal* and a contributor to *As the Wind Blows, Vol. 2*. Dr. Goldie lives in Chicago with her husband, Edward.

Learn more at askdrgoldiemd.com

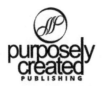

## CREATING DISTINCTIVE BOOKS
## WITH INTENTIONAL RESULTS

We're a collaborative group of creative masterminds with a mission to produce high-quality books to position you for monumental success in the marketplace.

Our professional team of writers, editors, designers, and marketing strategists work closely together to ensure that every detail of your book is a clear representation of the message in your writing.

### Want to know more?
Write to us at info@publishyourgift.com
or call (888) 949-6228

Discover great books, exclusive offers, and more at
**www.PublishYourGift.com**

Connect with us on social media

@publishyourgift